The International Library of Psychology

LUCIFER AND PROMETHEUS

Founded by C. K. Ogden

The International Library of Psychology

ANALYTICAL PSYCHOLOGY
In 12 Volumes

I	Studies in Analytical Psychology	*Adler*
II	Complex/Archetype/Symbol in the Psychology of C G Jung	*Jacobi*
III	Psychology of C G Jung	*Jacobi*
IV	Experiment in Depth	*Martin*
V	Amor and Psyche	*Neumann*
VI	Art and the Creative Unconscious	*Neumann*
VII	The Origins and History of Consciousness	*Neumann*
VIII	Jung's Psychology and its Social Meaning	*Progoff*
IX	Religion and the Cure of Souls in Jung's Psychology	*Schaer*
X	Conscious Orientation	*van der Hoop*
XI	Lucifer and Prometheus	*Werblowsky*
XII	The Secret of the Golden Flower	*Wilhelm*

LUCIFER AND PROMETHEUS

A Study of Milton's Satan

R J ZWI WERBLOWSKY

Introduction by C G Jung

ROUTLEDGE

First published in 1952 by
Routledge

Reprinted in 1999 by
Routledge
2 Park Square, Milton Park, Abingdon, Oxon, OX14 4RN

Transferred to Digital Printing 2007

British Library Cataloguing in Publication Data
A CIP catalogue record for this book
is available from the British Library

Lucifer and Prometheus
ISBN 0415-20948-X
Analytical Psychology: 12 Volumes
ISBN 0415-21124-7
The International Library of Psychology: 204 Volumes
ISBN 0415-19132-7

CONTENTS

INTRODUCTION

BY C. G. JUNG

The author has submitted his manuscript to me with the request that I should write a few words by way of introduction. As the subject of the book is essentially literary, I do not feel altogether competent to express an opinion on the matter. The author has, however, rightly discerned that although the problem of Milton's *Paradise Lost* is primarily a subject for literary criticism, it is, as a piece of confessional writing, fundamentally bound up with certain psychological presuppositions. Though he has only touched on these—at least in so many words—he has made it sufficiently plain why he has appealed to me as a psychologist. However little disposed I am to regard Dante's *Divine Comedy* or Klopstock's *Messiah* or Milton's *opus* as fit subjects for psychological commentary, I cannot but acknowledge the acumen of the author, who has seen that the problem of Milton might well be elucidated from that angle of research which is my special field of study.

For over two thousand years the figure of Satan, both as a theme of poetico-religious thinking and artistic creation, and as a mythologem, has been a constant psychological expression, having its source in the unconscious evolution of 'metaphysical' images. We should go very wrong in our judgement if we assumed that ideas such as this derive from rationalistic thinking. All the old ideas of God, indeed thought itself, and particularly numinous thought, have their origin in *experience*. Primitive man does not think his thoughts, they simply *appear* in his mind. Purposive and directed thinking is a relatively late human achievement. The numinous image is far more an expression of essentially unconscious processes than a product of rational inference. Consequently it falls into the category of psychological objects, and this raises the question of the underlying psychological presuppositions. We have to imagine a millennial process of symbol-formation which presses towards consciousness, beginning in the darkness of prehistory with primordial or archetypal images, and gradually developing and differentiating these images into conscious creations. The history of religion in the West can be taken as an illustration of this: I mean the historical development of dogma, which also includes the figure of Satan. One of the best-known archetypes, lost in the grey mists of antiquity, is the triad of gods. In the early centuries of Christianity it reappears in the Christian formula of the Trinity, whose pagan version is *Hermes ter unus*. Nor is it difficult to see that the great goddess of the Ephesians has been resurrected in the δεοτόκος. This latter problem, after lying dormant for centuries, came into circulation again with the dogma of the Immaculate Conception and, more recently, of the Assumption of the Virgin. The image of the mediatrix rounds itself out to almost classical perfection, and it is especially noteworthy that behind the solemn promulgation of the dogma there stands no arbitrary tenet of papal authority but an anonymous movement of the Catholic world. The numerous miracles of the Virgin which preceded it are equally autochthonous; they are genuine and legitimate experiences springing directly from the unconscious psychic life of the people.

I do not wish to multiply examples needlessly, but only to make it clear that the figure of Satan, too, has undergone a curious development, from the time of his first undistinguished appearance in the Old Testament texts to his heyday in Christianity. He achieved notoriety as the personification of the adverse principle of evil, though by no means for the first time, as we meet him centuries earlier in the ancient Egyptian Set and the Persian Ahriman. Persian influences have been conjectured as mainly responsible for the Christian devil. But the real cause of his differentiation into a separate figure is the conception of God as the *summun bonum*, which stands in sharp contrast to the Old Testament view and which, for reasons of psychic balance, inevitably requires the existence of an *infimum malum*. No logical reasons are needed for this, only the natural and unconscious striving for balance and symmetry. Hence very early on, in Clemens Romanus, we meet with the conception of Christ as the right hand and the devil as the left hand of God, not to speak of the Judaeo-Christian view which recognized two sons of God, Satan the elder and Christ the younger. The figure of the devil then rose to such exalted metaphysical heights that he had to be forcibly depotentiated, under the threatening influence of Manichaeism. The depotentiation was effected—this time—by rationalistic reflection, a regular *tour de force* of sophistry which defined evil as a *privatio boni* (the privation of good). But that did nothing to stop the belief from arising in many parts of Europe during the eleventh century, mainly under the influence of the Catharists, that it was not

God but the devil who had created the world. In this way the archetype of the imperfect demiurge, who had enjoyed official recognition in Gnosticism, reappeared in altered guise. (The corresponding archetype is probably to be found in the *cosmogonic jester* of primitive peoples.) With the extermination of the heretics that dragged on into the fourteenth and fifteenth centuries an uneasy calm ensued, but the Reformation thrust the figure of Satan once more into the foreground. I would only mention Jakob Boehme, who sketched a picture of evil which leaves the *privatio boni* pale by comparison. The same can be said of Milton. He inhabits the same mental climate. As for Boehme, although he was not a direct descendant of alchemical philosophy whose importance is still grossly underrated he certainly took over a number of its leading ideas, among them the specific recognition of Satan, who was exalted to a cosmic figure of first rank in Milton, even emancipating himself from his subordinate position as the left hand of God (the role assigned to him by Clement). Milton goes even further than Boehme and apostrophizes the devil as the true *principium individuationis*, a concept which had been anticipated by the alchemists some time before. To mention only one example: 'Ascendit a terra in coelum, iterumque descendit in terram et recipit vim superiorum et inferiorum. Sic habebis gloriam totius mundi.' (He rises from earth to heaven and descends again to earth, and receives the power of above and below into himself. Thus thou wilt have the glory of the whole world.) The quotation comes from the famous alchemical classic, the *Tabula Smaragdina*, attributed to Hermes Trismegistus, whose authority remained unchallenged for more than thirteen centuries of alchemical thought. His words refer not to Satan, but to the *filius philosophorum*, whose symbolism, as I believe I have shown, is identical with that of the psychological 'self'. The *filius* of the alchemists is one of the numerous manifestations of Mercurius, who is called 'duplex' and 'ambiguus' and is also known outside alchemy as 'utriusque capax'—capable of anything. His 'dark' half has an obvious affinity with Lucifer.

In Milton's time these ideas were very much in the air, forming part of the general stock of culture, and there were not a few Masters who realized that their philosophical stone was none other than the 'total man.' The Satan-Prometheus parallel shows clearly enough that Milton's devil stands for the essence of human individuation and thus comes within the scope of psychology. This close proximity, as we know, proved a danger not only to the metaphysical status of Satan, but to that of other numinous figures as well. With the coming of Enlightenment metaphysics as a whole began to decline, and the rift which then opened out between knowledge and faith could no longer be repaired. The more resplendent figures in the metaphysical pantheon had their autonomy restored to them practically untarnished, which assuredly cannot be said of the devil. In Goethe's *Faust* he has dwindled to a very personal *familiaris*, becoming the mere 'shadow' of the struggling hero. After rational-liberal Protestantism had, as it were deposed him by order of the day, he retired to the shadier side of the Christian Olympus as the 'odd man out', and thus, in a manner not unwelcome to the Church, the old principle reasserted itself: *Omne bonum a Deo, omne malum ab homine*. The devil remains as an appendix to psychology.

It is a psychological rule that when an archetype has lost its metaphysical hypostasis, it is identified with the conscious mind of the individual, which it influences and refashions after its own mind. And since an archetype always possesses a certain numinosity, the integration of the numen generally produces an inflation of the subject. It is therefore entirely in accord with psychological expectations that Goethe should dub his Faust a Superman. Nowadays this type extends beyond Nietzsche into the field of political psychology, and its incarnation in man has had all the consequences that might have been expected to follow from such a misappropriation of power.

As human beings do not live in airtight compartments, this infectious inflation has spread everywhere and given rise to an extraordinary uncertainty in morals and philosophy. The medical psychologist is bound to take an interest in such matters, if only for professional reasons, and so we witness the memorable spectacle of a psychiatrist introducing a critical study of Milton's *Paradise Lost*. Meditating upon this highly incongruous conjunction, I decided that I should best fulfil my obligations if I explained to the well-intentioned reader how and why the devil got into the consulting-room of the psychiatrist.

March 1951

ACKNOWLEDGEMENT

A SUMMARY of the argument of the present study is given in the Preface, so that this short prefatory note can limit itself to the customary ritual of publicly paying one's debts. As a matter of fact this act is often tantamount to a public proclamation of bankruptcy, but it has always been held nobler for the mind to make voluntary confession than to be found out by others. It is possibly for this reason that authors, eager to forestall their critical readers, have hit upon the idea of prefacing their books with lists of acknowledgements. Certainly the present writer is profoundly conscious of the truth that it is in our rare moments of original insight that more than ever we feel the easy yoke of our indebtedness to others.

As far as the literary criticism of *Paradise Lost* proper is concerned, the reader will notice that I have followed Professor Waldock's *Paradise Lost and Its Critics* almost to the point of plagiarism. As to the wider issues raised by Milton's poem, particularly in their theological and psychological bearings, I am deeply indebted to Professor G. Wilson Knight, especially to his *Chariot of Wrath*. I also wish to thank Messrs. Faber & Faber for their kind permission to quote extensively from the last-mentioned work.

Professor H. W. Häusermann of the University of Geneva watched the progress of this study, and helped with its final redaction and publication with a fatherly solicitude and severity. His untiring and encouraging sympathy, together with his scholarly and kind yet unsparing criticism, have repeatedly prevented me from making a still greater fool of myself. Much valuable criticism was also given by Professor R. Stamm and Dr. F.-C. Clavé.

It is a sad reflection that to acknowledge one's obligations is to be ungrateful towards all those whose names are not recorded or even forgotten. Our memory seems to be the most successful and incurable of all thieves; and much of what we regard as our own fond invention too often turns out to be a residue of previous reading or listening. Acknowledgements, bibliographies, footnotes and the like are therefore of doubtful value, and I shall limit myself to the names of them but for whom the present study would never have been written. These are Dr. Riwkah Schärf, of the C. G. Jung Institute for Analytical Psychology in Zürich, to whom I owe a great personal debt, in addition to that shared by all interested in the subject for her conclusive and classic study on the Satan in the Old Testament; Dr. Marie-Louise von Franz, of the same institute, who in the course of a few discussions gave me the clue to the themes elaborated in Chapters 2 and 3; and, last but not least, my great friend Henri van Praag, whose friendship and conversation are an unfailing source of wisdom and understanding, and a perpetual provocation to persevere in the quest for that truth which, according to St. Augustine, dwells *in interiore homine*.

To Professor Jung I would express at this place my profound and respectful thanks for his extreme kindness in examining the MS. and for the honour he has bestowed upon me by writing an Introduction. To attempt to thank him for more would be sheer presumption, but I hope that my study as such expresses what I owe to him. I am similarly indebted to Professor Kerényi, but I would not fail especially to put on record my profound gratitude for his reading through the whole MS. and expressing his agreement with its substance.

Mr. I. L. Palache has been of great assistance in preparing the MS. The Dean of St. David's, the Very Rev. C. Witton-Davies, has corrected the MS. and translated those foreign quotations which are not given in the original. If the defectiveness of my style and the multitude of faults have proved obdurate even to his correcting pen, it is certainly to the author's dishonour and not to his.

Finally I have taken leave to dedicate this thesis to my parents. Not so much, I would add, in the illusion that this would represent an adequate mark of gratitude, but rather in recognition of the sheer impossibility of rendering them even a fraction of what I owe to them.

Amsterdam
Summer 1951

PREFACE

A BOOK on Milton's Satan is not only about Milton, it is also about Satan. There were times when to write on the former would have been regarded as a matter of course, whilst the latter would have called for a modest apology. To-day the situation is, if not reversed, at least easier for a writer on matters diabolic. It is not the writers who have reintroduced the devil, but it is our present world which has forced them to take notice of him again. As a friend of mine once remarked: 'I don't know about angels, but I don't see how one can possibly doubt the devil.' Luther's advice to laugh at the devil *quia est superbus spiritus et non potest ferre contemptum sui* may do as an occasional exorcism, but is lamentably inadequate as a radical cure. We are living through times where evil has manifested itself with an almost revelation-like obtrusiveness and power. We have learned to understand the medieval legends about monks who, being vouchsafed a glimpse into hell, would never smile or speak again. The apocalyptic beast let loose[1] has become a reality to our generation, and nobody knows what is still ahead of us. It is understandable therefore that books on the devil have been on the increase lately. Edward Langton calls the last chapter of his study[2] 'The Return of Satan', giving as a recent example Professor C. E. M. Joad's *God and Evil*. We might add C. S. Lewis' *Screwtape Letters*, Denis de Rougemont's *La Part du Diable* and others. The Carmelite Fathers in France have edited a remarkable symposium on *Satan*.[3] The analytical psychology of Jung has already

1. It may be interesting to note that the occurrence of this incident from *Rev.* xx has been forecast for our times by a visionary of the last century. In the visions of Katharina Emmerich (d. 1824) one can read: 'In der Mitte [i.e. of hell] war ein Abgrund von Nacht, Luzifer ward gefesselt in diesen geworfen u. es brodelte schwarz um ihn. Es geschah alles dieses nach bestimmten Gesetzen, ich hörte dass Luzifer, wo ich nicht irre, 50 oder 60 Jahre vor dem Jahre 2000 nach Christus wieder auf eine Zeit lang solle freigelassen werden.' (*Das bittere Leiden unseres Herrn Jesu-Christi, nach den Betrachtungen der gottseligen Anna Katharina Emmerich* (ed. 1931), p. 311.)

2. *Satan: A Portrait. A Study of the Character of Satan through all the Ages* (1945).

3. Published as a special number of the *Revue Carmelitaine* (1948).

long insisted on bringing the devil and the problem of the shadow to the fore; mainly in connection with analytical treatment, but also, more recently, in theoretical research. It suffices here to mention Professor Jung's essay on the Trinity and Miss Schärf's stirring study on the Old Testament Satan.[4] If the attempts of this school have not yet borne much fruit, it is because we fear the devil's sight more than his activity, and because of a very understandable reticence to force open our 'whited sepulchres'. Novelists too are returning to the habit of introducing the devil, and using him as a *dramatis persona*. It may therefore be excused if one of the greatest and most towering Satans of literature is made the subject of a new study.

The problem is well known: Milton's Satan is somehow not satanic enough, his qualities are of a sort which defeats his satanic function in the poem. So much so that in due course the comparison with Prometheus was launched by the romantics, and has since then remained a constant feature in Miltonic criticism. Unfortunately however, this analogy, suggestive as it is, was never elaborated. It was rather vaguely understood, perhaps only meant, to convey a sense of the heroic at its limits, by pointing to the similarities in the situations of both heroes in their revolt against an order imposed by divine omnipotence; but that was all. Yet the figures of both Satan and Prometheus are interesting enough to warrant a closer inquiry into possible relationships.

But before proceeding with this inquiry I should like to point out that I am using these and similar terms throughout in the sense of C. G. Jung and his school. By 'figures' I thus mean mythological projections of the human *psyche*, in this case of the transpersonal collective unconscious, made up by one or more archetypes and expressive of various stages and levels of psychic development. Similarly the word 'relationships' denotes projections containing identical, related or similar archetypal features. All statements in this study concerning God, Satan, and similar concepts should be taken in that sense. I would have it understood, however, that this study is not primarily concerned with archetypes, and this term, when used, should not be taken in its restricted and accurate (and actually only permissible) sense. Consequently, I have refrained here from making the necessary distinctions[5]

4. It is difficult to overestimate the significance of Miss Schärf's study, both from a theological as well as from the psychological point of view. It is, so far as I can see, the only convincing theory of the Biblical Satan, and one may hazard the guess that it will remain so. I would take this opportunity to point out that Miss Schärf's main thesis is at the basis of the present study and forms an integral part of the argument of Chapter 4.

5. Cf. e.g., the second essay 'Bild, Gestalt und Archetypus' in K. Kerényi: *Niobe* (1949), as also the first chapter of the same author's *Die Antike Religion* (1940).

between archetype, myth, image, symbol, idea, and similar terms. The word is used here rather loosely to refer to the basic and supposedly universal preoccupations of humanity which are thought to inhere in the very structure of the soul, and of which the varieties of cultures with their different mythologies, imageries and concepts, are typical expressions. In other words, it is to a very large extent the *Kulturtypische* rather than the *Archetypische*[6] which will be our main concern here.

If Milton's Satan really exhibits a relationship with the Prometheus-figure, it ought to be worth our while to study him from this angle. The claim made in this study is that Milton's Satan in fact contains Promethean elements, and that these are the reasons for his powerful appeal—an appeal which has proved detrimental to the unity and purpose of the poem.

To substantiate this claim, a short account is given of the history and present state of *Paradise Lost* criticism, and an exposition of the poem's shortcomings, inconsistencies, and disharmonies. These preliminaries are all the more necessary, as our investigation will finally take us beyond the poem, and make us look for outside evidence. If there is any justification for such a method, it can only be that the poem itself, the line formed by its points of cleavage, serves as a finger-post indicating the direction in which we should transcend it.

This then is the limit to which literary criticism can take us. The reasons and realities responsible for the cleavage lie outside the province of literary criticism proper. Perhaps one should look for them in sociology, biography or psychology. Although it might be relevant, I have not attempted a *tiefenpsychologische* analysis of Milton's person (typological, animus-anima relation and the like) such as, e.g., Professor Jung has repeatedly done for Goethe.

Neither do I attempt here an analysis of the history and meaning of the Lucifer-myth. This has already been done, and is still being done by others, more capable and competent. Milton's personality will interest us in its bearing on Satan only. It is Miltonic psychology as the 'genetic' interpretation of Satan, whereas the 'structural' psychology of the latter will concern us only as mythology. My endeavour is simply to show that the realities behind the shortcomings of *Paradise Lost* are those of the human soul, or rather of the world as conceived by the human soul, and as expressed in such myths as that of Satan and Prometheus. It is my contention that the archetypal similarities between these myths led to contaminations of which the strange Satan of *Paradise Lost* is the result. Miltonic psychology is introduced only as far as necessary to describe the conditions and personal background of this

6. I owe both the distinction and the terms to Professor Kerényi.

'merger'. What ultimately matters is that Milton proved himself a great poet by bodying forth these realities and experiences.

The literary analysis of *Paradise Lost* reveals the dichotomy of Christian civilization in general as expressed in the ambivalence of such key-symbols as 'Power', the 'Kingdom', and the god-image itself. Particularly the latter undergoes a process of differentiation of far-reaching consequence. Whereas the original Hebrew civilization, based on the experience of a call and choice by God, could easily affirm civilization as god-willed, post-exilic development came increasingly under the influence of pagan, i.e., Greek and Persian[7] thought. This led in due course to a complete and fatal dissociation of spheres: good and evil, god and anti-god, power, that is to say action, versus inactivity and suffering, heaven and earth, spirit and matter, grace and nature, the kingdom of God and the World. As a consequence Satan becomes the sole power-exponent in this sublunar, post-lapsarian but pre-eschatological universe, and thus stands as the prototype of human civilizing effort. Already here we have an important archetypal relation with Prometheus.

But the relation goes deeper, for we must connect the Old Testament-New Testament polarity just described, with the wider problem of Biblical and Greek culture, and particularly with the idea of *hubris* which haunts the latter like a nightmare. As will be shown, *hubris* represents a logical and apposite concomitant of the sort of spirituality that developed in Greece, and of which Platonic idealism and Stoicism are typical examples.[8] Christianity, though an active agency in transmitting the Hebrew legacy to Europe, was nevertheless in many respects more Greek than Biblical. Though denouncing the Greek *ratio*, wisdom, and *hubris*, and preaching the prophetic message of humility and divine childhood, it yet shared the Greek impulse to soar too high, or rather to leave earth too far behind.

The sense of trespass and sin inherent in the dynamism of human life, which, to our modern consciousness is typically 'Christian', is in fact essentially Greek. This sense, unrelieved by a sense of calling (for that was a Jewish discovery), is expressed in the myth of Prometheus.

7. I ignore, for the present, the question of the relation between Greek and Persian thought. Cf. Jane Harrison, *Themis* (2nd ed. 1927), pp. 445–6, and part. p. 462, notes 1 and 5.

8. I would take this opportunity to enter a caveat against the many generalizations to be found in Chapters 2 and 3, particularly in the matter of Greek thought and culture. I am fully aware that the issues involved are far more complex than represented here. But it is not our purpose to give a full account of the various stages of development of Greek civilization, but to seize simply, even arbitrarily, on those aspects that bear on the Miltonic problem discussed here.

Prometheus is not only a hero, he is in the first place a sinner. We have here an attitude to culture whose parallel is not the Old Testament, but the Old Testament Apocrypha.

That these various modes of *prise de conscience*, these conflicting strands in our civilization, should clash in Milton's person, can easily be demonstrated. Both his biography and his poems bear witness to the extent to which he was obsessed by *hubris*: intellectually and morally. As is to be expected, the shadow of *hubris*, excessive sensuality, is not far away either. But equally marked was his sincere and profound Hebraism, or rather Old Testament-Christianity. In addition to this, his immense learning, classical, theological, and rabbinical, made him the predestined battling-ground for these contradictory forces. There is much to show that he was indeed the vessel of the wrath of this antinomy. In *Paradise Lost*, it would seem, these conflicts and contradictions are given a local habitation and a name.

It thus happens that Prometheus, the sinner and culture-hero, can be detected in the Satan of *Paradise Lost*. Milton's Satan has absorbed so many Promethean qualities that we are in danger of admiring him and sympathizing with him. Satan is in trespass and thus sinful; but at the same time he represents our (Greek and unregenerate) aspiration towards new and higher levels of existence, our human battle against heavy and indifferent odds.

This does not mean that there are identifiable literary connections between Prometheus and Satan, nor do I claim any influence of Aeschylos on Milton. All the argument wants to show is that the unconscious archetypal meaning or mythological contents of the Prometheus figure, is so near to that of Satan, that it could easily be absorbed by the latter, and that this absorption has in fact taken place to a remarkable degree in Milton's *Paradise Lost*.

There are of course many instances of antinomianism, and of too positive an appreciation of Satan in religious history. I have nevertheless desisted from mentioning these in connection with Milton. There seem to be no indications that Milton's Satan has anything to do with Gnostic beliefs and heresies. That the real trouble with Milton's Satan lies in his heavy Promethean charge is borne out by his vehement condemnation of civilization.

Milton's Satan is great because he has absorbed so many Promethean elements; and Prometheus is condemned because he is identified with Satan. What is involved in this mythological, or rather poetical amalgamation, will be discussed in Chapters 5 and 6. Unfortunately there is little synthesis in Milton's life and poetry. The burden of both appears to be that we should not *also* but *mainly* serve by standing and waiting.

Chapter One

HERO AND FOOL

It is one of the interesting characteristics of most human activities, that with the progress of time, developments and changes take place at an ever quicker rate. Miltonic criticism has been no exception to this rule. Whereas the 'romantic' critical tradition, culminating at the beginning of the twentieth century, could look back on more than a century of steady, albeit unequal growth, the first half of the twentieth century has already seen at least two significant revolutions. If dates must needs be assigned, we may consider Raleigh's *Milton* (1900) as the last great expression of the romantic tradition before the turning of the tide, which set in in 1917 with Greenlaw's now classic article, 'A Better Teacher than Aquinas'.[1] There followed a period of much scholarly activity, mainly in America and on the Continent, in the course of which a new Milton seemed to emerge: a somewhat depuritanized renaissance artist. Particularly the European group, headed by Professor Liljegren, did much to bring out the renaissance traits in Milton's character and art, and one of them, the 'diabolic' Mutschmann, undertook to lead the movement *ad absurdum* by pushing their methods and conclusions to fantastical extremes. The work of Professor Saurat, though lying outside these groups,[2] nevertheless tended to strengthen the impression of Milton as a bold, adventurous personality, a man whose basic emotions were a monumental pride and powerful egotism, and a thinker of terrible thoughts, who would drink heresies from any of the many 'turbid streams' of contemporary mystical and sectarian speculation. Meanwhile a new turning-point was reached when much detailed and patient, mainly American research had amassed overwhelming evidence of the traditional, conventional, and orthodox commonplaces embedded in almost every line of Milton. The dashing Satanist had given way to the conventional poet who would not say anything unless

1. In *Studies in Philology* (April 1917), xiv, 196–217.
2. Denis Saurat, *Milton, Man and Thinker* (1925), p. 342.

seventeen people had said it before,[3] and the pendulum has now gradually swung back to a definitely Christian, though not precisely puritan interpretation of Milton's poetry.

Ultimately all discussions of Miltonic problems in their wider sense are centred round *Paradise Lost*. For the purpose of this study, these will be taken notice of to the extent that they bear on the problem of Satan. For Satan too has had a sort of revival, ranging from sober academic survey to downright abuse and moderate defence. Obviously the appreciation of *Paradise Lost* generally, and of the vicissitudes of Satan in particular is dependent on, though not always identical with the critical movements outlined above. At times they run parallel, at other times they cut across each other. A detailed survey of *Paradise Lost* and Satanic criticism is unnecessary at this stage, as this will be done when we come to analyse more closely the problem of Satan.[4] It will suffice here to give a short list of some of the more important titles.

These are Dr. E. W. M. Tillyard's *Milton* (part iii) (1930), Mr. Charles Williams' introduction to the 'World's Classics' edition of the *English Poems* (1940), Mr. C. S. Lewis' *A Preface to Paradise Lost* (1942), Professor E. E. Stoll's 'Give the Devil his Due: a reply to Mr. Lewis' (1944),[5] Mr. G. Rostrevor Hamilton's *Hero or Fool? A Study of Milton's Satan* (1944), Professor S. Musgrove's article 'Is the Devil an Ass?'[6] and finally two recent studies, both of 1947: Professor A. J. A. Waldock's *Paradise Lost and its Critics* and B. Rajan's *Paradise Lost and the Seventeenth-century Reader*. There are of course many more authors and critics to be mentioned, and the above selection is not free from arbitrariness. Some of them will be mentioned later in the course of our analysis, others must be passed over, as Milton-criticism has grown so enormously that it is wellnigh impossible to do justice to every writer, unless one is prepared to convert one's study into a catalogue or another Milton bibliography.

Yet in spite of the formidable bulk and critical penetration of all that has been said and written about the Satan of *Paradise Lost*, there is still very much that has been left unsaid and unwritten. This is not due to any diabolic resistance on the part of Satan to having himself dismembered into his elements, analysed and critically re-examined. The far more diabolic reason is the lack of agreement as to who and what this Satan of the poem actually is. Ask ten critics to read through *Paradise Lost*, and then put to them the simplest and most fundamental of all questions: How does Satan strike you? and you will receive ten different

3. Cf. B. Rajan, *Paradise Lost and the Seventeenth-century Reader* (1947), p. 13 and pp. 12–13 for a bibliography of the more important publications on the subject.

4. Cf. pp. 4 ff.

5. *R.E.S.* xx 108–24.

6. *R.E.S.* xxi 302–15.

answers. It is to these answers, and to the simple question: How does Satan strike you? that the following sections of this chapter are devoted.

Largely, and therefore inaccurately speaking, there have been two main schools: the Satanists and the anti-Satanists. The latter can be subdivided into two not very sharply distinguished groups: those who loathe Satan as the originator or personification of Evil, and those who consider him a mean and contemptible fool. The Satanists too can be divided into perverse extollers of Satan and all he stands for, and into gallant and chivalrous opponents who feel bound in honour to pay homage to the Great Enemy's nobler qualities, his loyalty in leadership, fortitude in adversity, unflinching courage and splendid recklessness, in short, all the qualities usually comprehended by the adjective 'Promethean'.

Now the first interesting fact to be noted in this connection is that until Blake's *Marriage of Heaven and Hell* (about 1790), nobody ever appears to have been seduced by Satan's Promethean charms.[7] His greatness was recognized and admitted, not so much to magnify, let alone admire him, but to communicate the awareness that Satan was and is a redoubtable enemy, that the war in heaven was worthy of its protagonists and setting, and that the fall of the angels was no mean event. For the rest Satan was not regarded as particularly inspiring or fascinating. One knew of course that he was actually far worse than the Miltonic presentation of him, but this presentation was appreciated as tactful considerateness for the reader's Christian touchiness, 'A devil all made up of wickedness would be too shocking to any reader or writer'.[8] Already Addison had similarly praised Milton's delicacy of feeling: 'His [Satan's] sentiments . . . suitable to a created being of the most exalted and most depraved nature. . . . Amid those impieties which this enraged spirit utters . . . the author has taken care to introduce none that is not big with absurdity, and incapable of shocking a religious reader.'

Dryden's remark that Satan was the hero of *Paradise Lost*, can be left out of account here, as Dryden was thinking in terms of epic technique only. But Blake[9] was in deadly earnest with his 'revaluation of all values'.

In writing his remarks, Blake became the father of what is now broadly termed the romantic school of Miltonic criticism, a label which is used to cover the extreme attitudes of Blake and Shelley; in a more moderate form such nineteenth-century critics as Hazlitt, Landor,

7. Cf. pp. 25–6 for a discussion of this.

8. Newton's note to *Paradise Lost*, ii, 483.

9. See Appendix A.

Ruskin and Macauley;[10] Sir Walter Raleigh, whose *Milton* 'may fairly be said to represent the standard opinion of the romantic school';[11] and, according to Professor Musgrove,[12] also such modern critics as Mr. Hamilton, Professor Stoll, and Professor Waldock. Many other names might be added to that list: C. H. Herford, Lascelles Abercrombie,[13] and to mention but two more of the great Miltonic scholars, Denis Saurat, and, in a way, even Dr. Tillyard.

The anti-Satanist party is best represented by the late Mr. C. Williams, Mr. C. S. Lewis, and Professor Musgrove.[14] Their main line of attack consists in denying the Satanists' silent assumptions: that we may take the Satan of Books I and II at his face value; that we should give ourselves up to these primary impressions; and that we are allowed to forget for a while that Satan is unrelentingly wicked, nay, that he is Evil. Once these axioms are repudiated, and we start with 'a good morning's hate' of Satan, his appearances and speeches will be seen and heard in a different light. We shall then be able to see his wickedness and meanness, his cruelty, falseness and intellectual hollowness. As it is no far cry from intellectual hollowness to complete idiocy, it is no wonder that Mr. Lewis has taken this step too. After all Milton himself is often at pains to depict his Satan as ugly and repellent and 'big with absurdity'.

But before embarking on a more detailed analysis of these divergent Satan-appreciations, it will not be amiss to state clearly what at the bottom the whole controversy is actually about. As far as I can see, it boils down to two different questions, the one purely literary and historical, the other mainly psychological, both with reference to the primary issue already mentioned: 'How does Satan strike us?' The first question concerns the validity of any answer to the 'How does Satan strike us' as a relevant factor for *Paradise Lost* criticism. In other words, our own reactions, however closely argued and justified, can have no value for determining the meaning of the poem Milton wrote. In

10. Whose famous essay 'Milton' in the *Edinburgh Review*, lxxxiv (1825), was occasioned by the publication of the *Treatise*.

11. J. H. Hanford, *A Milton Handbook* (1927), p. 268. On the 'Satanism' of the romantics cf. also Professor Mario Praz, *The Romantic Agony* (1933), Chap. 2: 'The Metamorphosis of Satan.'

12. *Art. cit.*, p. 302.

13. 'It is surely the simple fact that if *Paradise Lost* exists for any one figure, that is Satan. . . . It is in the figure of Satan that the imperishable significance of *Paradise Lost* is centred; his vast unyielding agony symbolizes the profound antinomy of the modern consciousness.' (Quoted by Tillyard, *op. cit.*, p. 276.)

14. For reasons which will soon be evident, I do not mention Mr. Rajan in this connection.

order to do this, we must first find out what was the mental climate, the 'universe of discourse' out of which and for which *Paradise Lost* was written. Only when we are quite clear about this, may we proceed to examine the extent to which *our* own mental and emotional make-up, *our* range of experience and *our* scales of value are similar or dissimilar; and only when this has been satisfactorily done, can there be any talk of taking the further step of bringing in our own reactions. The second point concerns the various answers that can be given to the question 'How does Satan strike us?' irrespective of their critical validity. To put it differently: assuming that we admit the validity of the question, and consequently also the relevance of any answer to it, what are the possible responses to Milton's Satan? It is important to point out that these two problems are, as a rule, not kept properly apart. The ensuing confusion not only vitiates much of *Paradise Lost* criticism, but also makes it seem that often when the Satanist-anti-Satanist war appears to rage the heaviest, the parties concerned are actually talking about different things.

As a matter of fact, the Satanist position is simply the answer to the question 'How does Satan strike us?' When the question is thus uncritically put, and we allow ourselves to be overpowered by the sheer impact of Books I and II, the Satanist reaction is the only possible one, and as long as we are concerned with that question alone, any attempt at minimizing or denigrating the figure of Satan is bound to be a failure, notwithstanding all the subtle argument and clever dialectics employed to this end. This method and its failure are exhibited almost to perfection in Mr. C. S. Lewis's, in many respects admirable, *A Preface to Paradise Lost*, and to a lesser degree in Professor Mu - grove's article 'Is the Devil an Ass?' A short examination of these two important statements of the anti-Satanist case will clear the ground for a more comprehensive vision of Satan and of the role he play' in *Paradise Lost*.

Mr. Lewis has set himself the task of sweeping away all traditional misconceptions about *Paradise Lost* in general and about Satan in particular. The debunking campaign he has launched against Satan is the most thorough and cogently argued that has been made so far. Satan has been made the object of all Mr. Lewis' hair-splitting logic, persuasive charm and subtle irony, but unfortunately of none of his poetic feeling and artistic receptivity, of which he has given so much proof on other occasions. Cleverness is a virtue of very doubtful value. Far from solving any real problems, whether in theology, philosophy, and art (including poetry), it more often tends to obscure the truth, leading at its best to intellectual unauthenticity, at its worst to downright dishonesty.[15] Cleverness is Mr. Lewis' greatest pitfall, and vitiates much of his most brilliant work. Neither the problem of evil, nor that of pain,[16] can be adequately treated with logic-chopping. A point by point review of Mr. Lewis' contentions is superfluous here as, in addition to Professor Stoll's reply, this has been competently done by Mr. Waldock.[17] But the most convincing and decisive argument remains the poem itself, provided it is read with the ears and the heart, or rather with the 'nose', as the Dutch writer Menno ter Braak once put it, and not with the brain alone. Certainly, Satan is the Father of Lies and the Prince of Evil, he stands for pride, malice, folly, lust (his own or Milton's) and whatever else one wishes to saddle him with. No one would think of denying this, and all the king's horses and all the king's men, nay, even Blake himself, cannot make an antinomian or devil-worshipper of Milton. Yet it is equally true, that as the world goes, good and evil coexist everywhere. 'Good and evil we know in the field of this world, grow up together almost inseparably', says Milton in his *Areopagitica*, and to this rule his Satan is no exception. He has a host of fine qualities with which Milton and his readers must and do sympathize. It has often been said that Satan degenerates in the course of the poem.[18] To-day critics prefer to speak of 'degradation',[19] and defend its necessity, as well as that of the preceding inflation of Satan's worth, on grounds of epic technique and the requirements of the poem. But the bare fact is that the Mount Niphates speech is somehow felt as an abrupt change, and that all the subsequent degradation stands apart and fails to link up with the 'other' Satan. The first impressions are so strong that there is nothing in the poem that can successfully override them. The cue once given, it is past alteration as 'the whole has already been set and tuned to a different key'.[20] Of course Milton detests Satan and misses no opportunity to call him names, but this may be due precisely to the fact that he himself found the description wanting in a way which demanded some 'balancing'. What remains to be accounted for is

15. *The Screwtape Letters* (1942) abound of instances of Mr. Lewis' 'amusing' method of argument by insinuation, e.g., putting his personal dislikes into the mouth of the Devil. Mr. Lewis happens to prefer parochial to congregational worship. So the tacticians of hell are for propagating the latter. (Let. xvi, p. 81.)

16. C. S. Lewis, *The Problem of Pain* (1940).

17. I have not seen Mr. Waldock's *Mr. C. S. Lewis and Paradise Lost*, Australian Engl. Ass. (Sept. 1943), but I suppose its main contents to be reproduced in his *Paradise Lost and its Critics*.

18. Cf. Masson's article 'The Three Devils', etc., in *Fraser's Mag.* (Dec. 1844).

19. The term is already used by Stopford Brooke in a letter to Garnett, 1 Jan. 1830. It is to be found again with C. S. Lewis and in Professor Musgrove's article, and is convincingly applied by Mr. Waldock, *op. cit.*, Chap. 4, e.g. p. 83.

20. Waldock, *op. cit.*, p. 82.

why Milton could not help investing this 'Traitor Angel' and 'false fugitive with so much courage, loyalty, and steadfastness. Not to admit these qualities is blinding oneself to one of the major features of the poem and betraying 'eyes that see not and ears that hear not'.

When pressed logically, Satan involves himself in innumerable contradictions, but then, these contradictions are not supposed to be pressed logically. The very revolt and fall is an enormous contradiction and absurdity in itself, succinctly stated by Professor Stoll,[21] Basil Willey[22] and others: that we must picture a God 'omnipresent, omniscient, omnipotent and benevolent', yet at the same time, like Zeus, 'localized in heaven, subject to gross attacks from his enemies, and administering the universe in a manner which it taxed Milton's utmost energies to justify'. As Mr. Charles Williams has put it: 'Milton knew as well as we that Omnipotence cannot be shaken',[23] but this unquestionable truth tells rather against the myth itself than against Milton, who did the only thing a poet can do in such a case. He made us temporarily forget this incongruity. 'The conflict . . . is dramatically real in proportion as you assent to the illusion of equality which the poem communicates.'[24] But Mr. Lewis does not allow the poem to communicate *to him* any illusions.[25] So following in the footsteps of Mr. Williams, he calmly watches Satan's 'solemn antics' and pronounces a diagnosis of acute softening of the brain. To form a 'clear and distinct idea' about the background of Satan's rebellion is, of course, an *a priori* impossibility. To inquire into it is as nonsensical as to ask what was there before God created the world. Psychology is an empirical science dealing with postlapsarian minds. Milton had to pitch on something, as Sir Herbert Grierson has pointed out,[26] in order to get the traditional pride motive and his story going, so he pitched on the Exaltation of the Son.[27] Mr. Lewis is outraged that 'in the midst of a world of light and love, of

21. *Poets and Playwrights* (1930), pp. 279 ff.

22. *The Seventeenth-century Background* (1934), p. 252.

23. *Op. cit.*, p. xv.

24. Rajan, *op. cit.*, p. 96.

25. At times even God himself—unlike Mr. Williams and Mr. Lewis—almost seems a victim of poetic illusions. For in spite of his disdainful and unruffled calm and his superior irony, he once all but forgets to 'have his foes in derision' and to laugh 'at their vain designs and tumults vain'. *Paradise Lost*, v, 719–29. Here it is God who speaks and not Beelzebub, as in i, 130–2. And were it not for the commentators, the innocent reader would perhaps never notice that the whole speech is meant to be one sustained strain of irony!

26. *Milton and Wordsworth* (1937), p. 116.

27. Professor Grierson nevertheless underrates the significance of this choice. It is more than a peg to hang Satan's pride on. It belongs to the 'christocentric' setting of the whole poem, and gives a new dimension to the Messiah's conflict with the Devil, and to his ultimate victory.

song and feast and dance, he could find nothing to think of more interesting than his own prestige'.[28] So would we all have been, had things happened in Dante's *Paradiso*.[29] As the story stands in Book V of *Paradise Lost*, we respond differently. God's speech is domineering, provocative, and dictatorial:

. . . him who disobeyes
Mee disobeyes, breaks union, and that day
Cast out from God and blessed vision, falls
Into utter darkness, deep ingulft, his place
Ordaind without redemption, without end.

P.L. v. 611–15

As Professor Wilson Knight has bluntly expressed it, it really is Messiah who starts all the trouble. Why God's threat and challenge 'where nothing but God's courteous consideration for his faultless subjects was needed'?[30] And once 'Satan is granted his motive, so must he be his own point of view'.[31] When Satan makes his momentous choice 'Evil be thou my Good' (*P.L.* iv. 110) Mr. Lewis thinks that Satan's level of intelligence has sunk below zero, as this is tantamount to asserting 'Nonsense be thou my sense'. I wonder whether Mr. Lewis has ever thought of expounding *Isaiah* v. 20: 'Woe unto them that call evil good, and good evil; that put darkness for light, and light for darkness; that put bitter for sweet, and sweet for bitter!' in a similar way, to wit that the prophet reproached the Israelites with sinning against logic as their only perversion. Mr. Lewis' criticism really amounts to an inversion of the mock-heroic method. 'He treats the superhuman in the light of commonsense', thus making 'personified self-contradiction' of Satan's passionate paradoxes.[32] One of the most powerful moments in *Paradise Lost* is Satan's agony at the sight of Adam and Eve 'Imparadis't in one anothers arms', as this brings home to him in a tormenting flash of insight what it means to be in hell, 'where neither joy nor love' (iv. 505–10). Mr. Lewis, I suppose, would reply here too: 'What do you mean by saying that we have lost love? There is an excellent brothel round the corner.'[33] This is worse than disgusting, it is unfair.

Yet even in this Mr. Lewis is not alone. In point of fact, the first to start hitting Satan below the belt was Milton himself. Professor Waldock has given a lucid and penetrating analysis of Milton's tech-

28. *Op. cit.*, p. 94.
29. Cf. Waldock, *op. cit.*, p. 73.
30. G. Wilson Knight, *Chariot of Wrath* (1942), p. 130.
31. E. E. Stoll, *art. cit.*, p. 112.
32. *Ibid.*, pp. 113–14.
33. *Op. cit.*, p. 103.

nique of dealing with Satan on two different levels.[34] The first may be called that of description, demonstration or exhibition, the second that of allegation or commentary. Milton is somehow aware of the threat his own Satan is becoming to his purpose. He therefore supplies his poem with a running commentary. Now whenever Satan makes one of his spirited and impressive appearances, and Milton tries to take him down a peg by quickly adding a nasty remark, we possess, *prima facie*, no criterion by which to decide which of the two conflicting presentations we ought to regard as more authoritative and final. The one infallible guide (infallible in spite of all attempts to discredit it as subjective, arbitrary and the like) is the reader's emotive response. Poetry is read and appreciated because—thank God—we still can distinguish between the heart-beat of genuine poetry, the fullness of a poet's life, and mere façade-poetry, where part only of the author's mind usurps the poet's gift to express itself. I have already referred earlier to Milton's habit of first ennobling his Satan and then calling him names, and it is with reference to this practice that Mr. Waldock is right in speaking of 'literary cheating'. 'Using the method of allegation, Milton can produce a trump card whenever he wishes. We have no defence against such tactics except . . . to take due note of what is going on and to decline to play when the trump has appeared too obviously from Milton's sleeve.'[35] A few examples may serve to illustrate this point.

Of all the many speeches in *Paradise Lost*, Belial's in the infernal council,[36] is one of the most sensible, sober and realistic. It is precisely what one would wish to hear from any responsible statesman. But Milton apparently dislikes such cowardice, preferring black and tan. So Belial is snubbed:

> *Thus* Belial *with words cloath'd in reasons garb*
> *Counsel'd ignoble ease, and peaceful sloath,*
> *Not peace* . . .
>
> *P.L.* ii. 226–8

Already Addison had praised this 'agreeable variety' in the description of the infernal party. 'Belial lewd and luxurious, now slothful and timorous, preferring to be miserable rather than not to be.' It may have escaped Milton and Addison that to prefer to be miserable rather than not to be is sound Biblical doctrine: *Ecclesiastes* ix. 4: 'for a living dog is better than a dead lion'. The passage is really worthy of Mr. Lewis: not 'reasonable' but clothed in reason's garb, not abstention from useless war but ignoble ease, no peace but peaceful sloth.

34. *Op. cit.*, pp. 77–81. 35. *Ibid.*, p. 81. 36. *P.L.*, ii. 119–225.

Satan's offer to undertake alone the perilous reconnaissance flight to the new world certainly shows a noble conception of leadership. It is far superior to its counterpart, Christ's offer to act as ransom for fallen man. Milton is apparently quite unaware how much is detracted from the greatness of Christ's sacrifice by his smug certainty of success and triumph.[37] But to detract from Satan's nobility, Milton had consciously and *deliberately* to cast aspersions at his motives.[38]

One would suppose that Lucifer, before becoming Satan, shared the habits and activities of the other good angels: adoring God and shouting Hallelujah. But no, he is severely rebuked by Gabriel for his pre-lapsarian virtues:

> . . . *thou sly hypocrite, who now wouldst seem*
> *Patron of liberty, who more than thou*
> *Once fawn'd, and cring'd, and servilly ador'd*
> *Heav'ns awful Monarch?*
>
> *P.L.* iv. 957–60

Professor Waldock calls this a 'high-handed piece of unsupported calumny'. I rather suspect that Milton, slightly off his track, gives away his real opinion (and, incidentally, that of many of his readers) as to what we should think about the revivalling crowd in heaven, who 'lowly reverent . . . bow and to the ground with solemn adoration . . . cast Thir Crowns' (*P.L.* iii. 349–52), as compared to the dashing self-reliance of Satan and his crew.

There are more of these contradictions, though some are less glaring because more purely literary. In Book IX, 27–41 Milton scoffs at the chivalric epic, whilst Michael plays the role of a St. George in a pseudo-Arthurian heaven. Temples and palaces, symbolizing the contemptibility of earthly magnificence, are raised in hell, by the same architect who had already previously built them in heaven.[39] Similarly we learn that Mammon, the first to dig for gold and to propagate the practice, had already had ample opportunity in heaven to give evidence of his weakness.[40] Apparently gold and the other splendours of heaven should be despised down here as the vanities of earth. It is inadequate to retort that precisely this corruption of good into evil is one of the poem's main themes. It is rather one of the unavoidable traps every poet falls into when he has to deal with good and evil. He has to choose aesthetic values and their current symbols: beauty, riches, majesty and the like, and to apply them to the good and holy. Otherwise he would fail to 'moralize his song' and would betray the avowed moral purpose

37. *P.L.*, iii. 242–59 ff.
38. *P.L.*, ii. 466–73.
39. *P.L.*, i. 732 ff.
40. *P.L.*, i. 680–2.

of his poetry. Similarly he would like to attribute horror, ugliness and repulsiveness to sin and evil. But then he would overlook the most conspicuous and also the most agonizing characteristic of evil, its powerful fascination and attractive beauty. How then are we to represent the train of the seven deadly sins if not doubly, in two different forms? In this respect too Spenser was a great teacher. His descriptions of evil are alternately disgusting and alluring. This dilemma is beautifully brought out by Milton's allegory of sin. She is 'Woman to the waste, and fair' but ends 'foul in many a scaly fould . . . a Serpent arm'd with mortal sting';[41] she is a 'Snakie Sorceress', Satan confessing that he never saw 'sight more detestable'. The break begins with l. 746:

> *Hast thou forgot me then, and do I seem*
> *Now in thine eye so foul, once deemd so fair.*
>
> *P.L.* ii. 747–8

From that point onward we get used to her as 'shining heav'nly fair' (l. 757) and endowed with 'attractive graces' (l. 762). It is absurd when Professor Musgrove,[42] arguing that Satan's degradation begins at Hell-Gate, finds evidence for this not only in our surprise when learning of his incest and dalliance, but in his throwing away all dignity by calling this foul Scylla his 'fair daughter'. The truth is that she *is* fair and must be, quite simply because she is sin. Not only Satan calls her 'Fair Daughter' (x. 384) but, in accordance with the principles outlined, also the poet himself: '. . . Sin, his faire Inchanting Daughter' (x. 352–3).

Even the anti-Satanists have to admit that Mr. Lewis's analysis is a critical aberration, and Professor Musgrove is far more moderate and cautious in his essay. Satan, he admits, is neither an idiot nor a nincompoop, and anyway, 'the intellectual impression is only part of . . . any poetic experience'.[43] If we overlook Satan's initial grandeur and fail to be stirred by it '*against our reason and against our will*', we are missing the titanic proportions of the struggle between good and evil.[44] But for the rest we must see the Satan of *Paradise Lost* as one character, and once we start with a 'good morning's hate' of him, and keep the whole concept, including his wickedness and intellectual rottenness, firmly in mind, we shall remain immune against the danger of upholding the initial impressions of Books I and II against the subsequent denigration. This sounds all very reasonable until we read the poem and try to

41. *P.L.* ii. 650–3, 724, 745. For the image as such cf. Spenser's Error and Echidna, *Faerie Queene*, Bk. I, C. i, St. 14 and Bk. VI, C. vi, St. 10, and Hesiod's *Theogony*, 298.

42. *Art. cit.*, p. 306. 43. *Ibid.*, p. 314. 44. *Ibid.*

match its impressions against some of Mr. Musgrove's arguments. It is certainly true that we start any book about a well-known character with presumptions. Even such an outspoken 'Satanist' as Mr. Hamilton begins with asserting that Satan should be approached *with* prejudice, and that we should not start by throwing our moral sense overboard.[45] One might even say that the importance of these presumptions increases proportionately with the dignity and celebrity of the character in question. It is equally true that these presumptions need not be expressly stated, but—and here comes the snag—they must be felt throughout. And this is not the case with Milton's Satan. His splendour simply overrides our consciousness of his evil. And God's infinite love is equally presumed but not felt! Professor Stoll is severely taken to task for making good his point by quoting almost exclusively from Books I and II. But one should pause to think for a moment why Professor Stoll has been tempted to do so. May it not be because the (admittedly partial) aspects of Satan to be found there, sound more authentic and convincing? Even if it is true that the Romantic critics 'start at the wrong end', their intuition did not come to them *ex nihilo*. It came from certain passages in *Paradise Lost*!

Of course they can be reproached with one-sided interpretation of these passages, stressing what Satan says to the exclusion of what he does.[46] 'In a narrative poem like *Paradise Lost* one must judge—as *mutatis mutandis* in a novel—not merely by a character's opinion of himself, but by other people's opinion of him, and by his actions as well as his sufferings. After all, he may be a liar, as Satan patently is'[47] and 'one wonders if in real life such critics accept every man's proclaimed valuation of himself'.[48] But one wonders too whether Professor Musgrove does not know that in an epic, as *mutatis mutandis* in a drama, the speech, viz., the dramatic soliloquy, is a conventional method of description and exposition, in no way less essential than the action. And when the two are so incompatible, there must be a reason for it, or rather for the fact that the one is so very much more convincing. And who, after all, are the 'other people' whose authoritative opinion we should take into consideration? Abdiel perhaps?

There is no use in trying to dodge the unpleasant facts. Even when making allowances for our own modern 'egalitarian or even antinomian' preconceptions, there still remains an undigestible lump of

45. *Op. cit.*, p. 8.

46. Musgrove, *art. cit.*, p. 303. This expression of Prof. Musgrove is very inaccurate. Actually in his degradation-speeches Satan sounds mean and hollow, whereas in his great moments he also acts greatly.

47. *Ibid.*, p. 304.

48. *Ibid.*, p. 303.

emotional disharmony in the poem, which Mr. Lewis, though aware of it,[49] is determined to make light of and to explain away. Milton may have had to endow Satan with some magnificence, as otherwise only a moron would have been left instead of the Archrebel, but what matters is that Milton *succeeded* so uncannily well! He may moreover have intended all his readers to be as astute as Mr. Lewis, but here again the fact is that Milton has grossly overrated his reading public. Finally Prof. Musgrove is trapped into preaching, and what he preaches is bad literary criticism and worse theology. He believes that not even the unregenerate man in us should thrill at Satan's grandeur, because (and this is the great discovery) 'Satan is only grand in Hell. . . . Evil can seem magnificent—against a background of evil, for evil is essentially false'.[50] The trouble with *Paradise Lost* is that Satan's grandeur is poetically real, and the trouble with the world is that Evil too is so solidly, so essentially real!

I do not see how one can escape Professor Waldock's conclusion that a great split runs through the poem, that the *Paradise Lost* Milton meant is not quite the one that he wrote, and that this is due 'to the radical ambiguity of what the poem asserts on the one hand, and what it compels us to feel on the other'.[51] Whether it is God who cannot speak twelve consecutive lines without antagonizing us, or Paradise and Heaven which simply bore us, or the sheer impossibility of showing the necessary horror at Adam's fall,[52] or of grasping the difference between pre- and post-lapsarian sex-behaviour, the poem continually asks for incompatible responses. 'In reading *Paradise Lost* we must not always expect to find that Milton's intention is perfectly matched by his performance—that what he meant to do in any given case has always its exact counterpart in what he did. Similarly . . . we must not always expect to find that what he has done is perfectly matched by his *theory* of what he has done.'[53] And with more direct reference to Satan: 'In a sense Milton's central theme denied him the full expression of his deepest interests. It was likely, then, that as his really deep interests could not find outlet in his poem in the right way, they might find outlet in the wrong way. And to a certain extent they do; they find vents and safety-valves often in inopportune places. Adam cannot give Milton much scope to express what he really feels about life: but Satan is there, Satan gives him scope. And the result is that the balance is somewhat disturbed. . . .'[54] This may be due in great part to the fact that, in the words of Professor W. P. Ker: 'Satan has all the heroism to himself, all the contending strength', but it is a fact which determines

49. *Op. cit.*, p. 77. 50. *Art. cit.*, p. 304. 51. Waldock, *op. cit.*, p. 143.
52. See pp. 20–1. 53. Waldock, *op. cit.*, p. 25. 54. *Ibid.*, p. 24.

the whole climate of the poem. Reviewing Mr. Lewis' *Preface*, Mr. B. A. Wright wrote:[55] '... the fact remains that Satan, though not the hero, is yet the most heroic figure in the poem. Mr. Lewis does not squarely face this fact, which is at bottom the romantic error.' Perhaps Mr. Wright ought to have said the 'romantic intuition'. Mr. Lewis has provided critics with an excellent criterion: 'The first qualification for judging any piece of workmanship from a corkscrew to a cathedral is to know what it is—what it was intended to do and how it is meant to be used.'[56] I think it is clear that Mr. Lewis' own conditions are not fulfilled by Satan, though of course that may be part of his wickedness. He simply does not do what he was intended to do, and is he not then, according to that very criterion, a bad piece of workmanship?

Awareness of this state of affairs is the basis of the Satanist interpretation. The tenets of this school are too well known to need repetition here.[57] They are inspired by a strong sensibility to the poetic reality of Satan's grandeur and magnificence, a grandeur which is not matched poetically by God, his angels, and the Messiah himself. It is unnecessary to prove this assertion by quotations, as these would amount to a reprint of a great part of *Paradise Lost*. The Satanist case obviously lends itself too easily to exaggerations, and then one either rushes to extremes, or one tries to make clear-cut distinctions between Milton's heart and his head, the poet and the believer, the great heretic and the great Puritan.[58] Whatever the value of Blake's remarks—and it is great indeed, as we shall see—the most satanic Satanist would not dream of considering them as a complete and sufficient statement of the facts about *Paradise Lost*. In that sense a Satanist school simply does not exist, or if it does, nobody belongs to it. Milton was for one no antinomian, and I would draw attention to the fact that Professor Stoll, one of the so-called modern Satanists, was about the only one who during the heydays of the Renaissance Milton insisted on the essentially puritan character of the poet. It is agreed by everyone that Satan is not only condemned, but actually degraded in the poem, and there is no need to follow here in detail this process, culminating in what Professor Waldock[59] calls the 'cartoon scene' of Book X, 418–570. It should however be mentioned here, that even the more recent and extremely moderate defenders of Satan at times allow their admiration to trick

55. *R.E.S.* xx (1944,) 83. 56. *Op. cit.*, p. 1.

57. Cf. p. 3 for Blake. Shelley and Sir W. Raleigh will be mentioned in another context. Cf. p. 47.

58. Cf. p. 76.

59. *Op. cit.*, pp. 91–2. The same process is also described by Mr. Musgrove and Mr. Rajan.

them into strange errors of interpretation of otherwise simple and unequivocal passages. This unfortunately makes some of their soundest and soberest analyses look partial and prejudiced. One of the most notorious examples is Satan's speech, *Paradise Lost* iv. 358–92. Here certainly Mr. Lewis and Mr. Musgrove are right, and Sir W. Raleigh,[60] Professor Stoll, Mr. Hamilton and Mr. Empsom[61] are wrong.

> . . . *whom my thoughts pursue*
> *With wonder, and could love, so lively shines*
> *In them Divine resemblance . . . etc.*
>
> *P.L.* iv. 362–4

does certainly not mean that Satan loved his prospective victims, as little as his description of himself as

> *no purpos'd foe*
> *To you whom I could pittie thus forlorne*
> *Though I unpittied*
>
> *Ibid.* 373–5

means that he pitied them. Similarly the lines

> *And should I at your harmless innocence*
> *Melt, as I doe, . . . etc.*
>
> *Ibid.* 388–9

bear the stamp of dishonesty and hollowness. Lines 375–81 ff.

> . . . *League with you I seek,*
> *And mutual amitie so streight, so close,*
> *That I with you must dwell, or you with me*
> *Henceforth; my dwelling haply may not please*
> *Like this fair Paradise, your sense, yet such*
> *Accept your Makers work; he gave it me*
> *Which I as freely give; . . . etc.*

reveal an abysmal cruelty, and are perhaps the direct inspiration of the final lines of *Screwtape Letters* Nos. xxii and xxxi.[62] Nevertheless, the speech is not quite as simple and unproblematical as Mr. Lewis and Professor Musgrove try to make it, and I rather incline to Professor Waldock's view that even here Milton is caught unawares, and charge his words with more power than he actually intended to do.

60. *Op. cit.*, pp. 137–8.
61. *Some Versions of Pastoral* (1935), p. 168. Surely the 'traditional' interpretation of these lines as the acme of brutal irony, is the only possible one.
62. *The Screwtape Letters*, pp. 115, 156, 160.

But in spite of these errors, we have no right 'to underestimate the intuition of Burns, Blake, Shelley, Byron, Coleridge, Landor, Racine and Chateaubriand, Hazlitt and Ruskin'.[63] Granting this, there is no further need to haggle about details, and to quarrel whether Dr. Tillyard has not gone far enough or whether Mr. Hamilton has gone too far, and as the rest of critical clap-trap may go. It is also irrelevant to our present purpose whether we believe with Professor Waldock that there are actually two different Satans in *Paradise Lost*, the Mount Niphates speech making no mere change but a definite break, or whether we agree with Mr. Musgrove and B. Rajan that Satan is one poetic whole throughout the twelve books of the poem. What does matter is, that shorn of its excrescences, the Satanist interpretation agrees with our response, which is not *our* response only, as, in the words of Professor Stoll, 'it is . . . quite impossible that for not much less than three centuries the readers of Milton should, in the mere matter of the imaginative and emotional impression of his "glorious fiends" have been so prodigiously mistaken'.[64]

In combating the Satanist school, the only scientific and fruitful procedure is to put the historical question alluded to earlier. Are we to allow our impressions of *Paradise Lost*, justifiable as they may be in themselves, to exert any influence on the statements we make about it? Can we legitimately and validly argue from our twentieth-century responses to the poem Milton wrote and Thomas Ellwood read? This question was raised on what seems to me so far the highest level in Miltonic criticism by Mr. Rajan, and a review of this important study is therefore indispensable.

In fact Mr. Rajan's point, once it has been made, seems so obvious and self-evident that one is surprised it has not been made earlier. As he himself writes, he is trying to do for Milton what is to-day commonplace in Elizabethan scholarship,[65] and it is a rather distressing symptom of the state of affairs in Miltonic research that a book like Mr. Rajan's has had to come forth at this time of the day. I think nobody would disagree with Mr. Rajan's thesis that the beginning of all wisdom is to consider a poem in its proper background, to try to understand the values, presumptions, modes of thought and feeling the poet *and his readers* (to whom the poem is, after all, addressed) bring to their experiences. Applying these rather vague and obvious generalities more concretely to the problem of Satan, we must ask: What did Satan mean to seventeenth-century readers? We shall discover then that Raleigh's alternative, Fool or Hero (taken up by Mr. G. R. Hamilton), is extremely misleading, because 'given certain ethical systems Satan is ultimately

63. Stoll, *art. cit.*, p. 114. 64. *Ibid.*, p. 124. 65. *Op. cit.*, p. 17.

heroic, given others, he is ultimately farcical'.[66] Similar to Professor Musgrove's good morning's hate of Satan, we must recognize that with Milton's contemporaries the devil was the Great Enemy, that he was consequently set against a background of 'unremitting hostility', and that the main response to him would be one of fear. Satan's grievances and complaints we must regard as specious, because none of Milton's contemporaries could have taken them seriously.[67] As Mr. Lewis has said: 'In the midst of a world of light and love, of song and feast and dance, he could find nothing to think of more interesting than his own prestige.' 'The heroic qualities which Satan brings to his mission, the steadfast hate, the implacable resolution . . . are qualities not to be imitated or admired. . . . The sympathy for Satan which the poetry imposes, the admiration it compels for his Promethean qualities, are meant to be controlled by this sort of moral reaction . . . the conflict is neither Promethean nor farcical. It is dramatically real in proportion as you assent to the illusion of the equality which the poem communicates.'[68] Satan must thus be conceived as a poetic, not as a cosmic force. At variance with Mr. Hamilton's conclusion 'that the poet had his reasons of which the Puritan knew nothing, that the Satan created by Milton's imagination was nobler and more admirable than the devil conceived by his intellect',[69] Mr. Rajan contends that 'Milton's heart was not at variance with his head . . . and his Satan . . . is . . . on the whole what he intended him to be'.[70]

Mr. Rajan's argument seems valid and impeccable as far as it goes. The trouble is that it does not go very far. The problem of the insufficiency of Mr. Rajan's attitude is related to the wider issue of the significance of literary-historical and -sociological research for the business of literary criticism proper. There is no doubt but the more we learn about the background of a work of art, the more certain, guided, and circumspect our appreciations will be. But the more usual result of this preoccupation with sources, backgrounds, popular doctrines, current traditions and what not, is the loss of the awareness that all this necessary research ought to be regarded, in the last resort, as the *ancilla* of literary criticism. One may almost speak here, with a slight variation of the Latin proverb, of *propter studium studendi perdere causas*. When I read *Antony and Cleopatra*, I am not interested in North's Plutarch. But I need Plutarch's description of Cleopatra's barge in order to understand what Shakespeare has done here, and to gain an other-

66. *Op. cit.*, pp. 94 ff.

67. *Ibid.*, p. 102. But cf. the end of this chapter, pp. 25–6, for a discussion of this point.

68. *Ibid.*, pp. 95–6. 69. Cf. Hamilton, *op. cit.*, p. 11. 70. Rajan, *op. cit.*, pp. 104 ff.

wise inaccessible insight into the nature of Shakespeare's poetry. It thus happens that 'in too full a revulsion, we may find ourselves asking what the proper study of literary mankind may be, if not precisely that "literary form", that "rapturous expression" and the kind of heart and blood which Milton's epic gave to the traditions'.[71] I am afraid I do not know why Mr. Martin qualifies this revulsion as 'too full', when in point of fact it is not nearly full enough. As far as Milton is concerned, this can best be illustrated by McColley's monumental essay 'Paradise Lost'[72] which is the standard repository of all the available evidence that both the theme and its treatment are conventional, orthodox, and commonplace. Even apparent deviations from the strict line of orthodoxy are shown to go back on traditions of their own. Thus what is most badly needed is 'some modifications of the often repeated statement that the Satan of *Paradise Lost* was the creation of Milton. The poet made Satan, as he made all other things in the epic, more magnificent, more compelling, than did his contemporaries'.[73] I am sure nobody has ever thought of enriching our understanding of such a line as: *Nymphs and shepherds, dance no more*, of which A. E. Housman[74] said that it could draw tears, with the comment that Milton did not coin here any new words, but just used the good old English vocabulary, only arranging the words in a 'more magnificent and compelling' manner than others. The example is not quite as silly as it may appear at first sight. No poet writes on a *tabula rasa*, and creativity involves among other things the capacity to select in a very peculiar way among given elements. It is not our purpose here to investigate the relation between creativeness, selectivity, originality and inventiveness and to determine the various degrees in which they are present in the various poets. But by and large this creative selectivity is one of the main elements of all poetic activity, and this holds true for the choice of words, as well as, in different manners, for the other levels of composition.

Discussing the 'pessimism'[75] which Dr. Tillyard regards as one of the hidden themes of *Paradise Lost*, Mr. McColley avows that he can find few traces of it, except, of course, the commonplaces. Nevertheless 'the tonal shading and treatment the poet has given these commonplaces is, of course, another matter, and may support the interpretation that *Paradise Lost* is the pessimistic creation of a disillusioned poet'.[76] That this 'aside' may contain the main problem, is simply ignored.

71. L. C. Martin: 'Shakespeare, Lucretius and the Commonplaces', *R.E.S.* xxi (1945), 174–5.

72. Grant McColley, 'Paradise Lost', *Harvard Theological Review*, xxxii (1939).

73. *Art. cit.*, p. 232.

74. *The Name and Nature of Poetry*, (1940), p. 46.

75. Cf. p. 65.

76. *Art. cit.*, p. 234.

But let us come back to Satan. Having shown that all the details of the fall, hell and the infernal council are conceived and worked out along conventional lines, Mr. McColley addresses himself to Satan. 'The last and greatest of the angels in *Paradise Lost* is Satan, a character long inspiring to both layman and scholar. Generally known as the creation of Milton, he has also been described as the poet himself, and as a personality so powerful that his creator was forced to dismiss him from the stage. *Such interpretations contain much that is true, but it remains a fact that the Satan of Books I and II, V–VI is basically a conventional and orthodox figure.*'[77]

There is no reason why we should not have it the other way round: 'Though there may be much that is true in the insistence on the conventional and orthodox elements in Satan, yet it remains a fact that he is essentially a creation of Milton.' It all depends on what we are looking for, and what we regard as more relevant to the problem of the poem and of its significance. It is one thing to state with St. Thomas that Lucifer was bright and glorious, sharing to a certain extent even the attributes of the Trinity, that he now continues steadfast and implacable in his hate and evil, and the like, and quite another to make these beliefs poetically so real, that they simply upset all balance!

The law that differences in quantity at a certain point change into differences in quality, is borne out by Satan. He has been endowed with so much greatness, heroic energy, and other virile virtues, that he becomes a different being which has to be considered in its own right. But even this is not enough. As has already been remarked earlier,[78] a split runs through the poem. The responses it demands are contradictory, because the actual poetic data to which we respond are not identical with our opinion about them, that is to say with the data to which we think we *ought* to respond. This means that we have here more than a mere case of quantity turning into quality. The 'positive' aspects of Satan are somehow as real and fundamental as our condemnation of him. Of course Mr. Rajan is right in maintaining that Satan is a poetic force, and that all sorts of elements have been fused into this 'aesthetic whole'. What remains to be explained is the failure of this fusion, and the power, insistence and obstrusiveness of the Promethean element, the fact, in short, that Milton selected it with all its 'charge', apparently blind to the consequences of this impossible combination. One of these consequences is that the average reader feels unable to agree with Mr. Rajan when he says that 'He [Milton] may justify God's ways, but he does not celebrate them'. It rather seems to be the other

77. *Art. cit.*, p. 198. Italics are mine.

78. Cf. p. 13.

way. Milton does celebrate God's ways in solemn, incantatory strains, but he does not succeed greatly in justifying them.[79]

Why did Milton so grievously fall short in his treatment of the Love-Mercy theme? and why is the Satan worked into the 'poetic whole', the Promethean one? and why, finally, does Mr. Rajan, after expounding to us what Milton's verse was supposed to do, and asserting rather half-heartedly that Milton's Satan was 'on the whole what he intended to make him', wistfully admit: 'But Milton's verse is not equal to the occasion'?[80]

Why not? Certainly not because Milton was unable *qua* poet to find a way of expressing what he intended to express. When we make full allowance for the seventeenth-century frame of mind, and discount everything our own different mental and emotional make-up brings to the poem, there still remains a considerable residuum of contradictions, glaring inconsistencies, and inequalities of poetical reality-levels (poetry too has its ontology!).

An interesting example of this, which incidentally illustrates in a nutshell all the confusion in and about *Paradise Lost*, is the story of Adam's fall. To try to define in so many words the nature of the fall, is a manifest absurdity. When Mr. Green,[81] M. Denis Saurat, Mr. Williams, Mr. Lewis, Dr. Tillyard and others have had their say about Adam and Eve: failure of intellect, failure of will, passion, injured merit, murder, pride, sensuality, uxoriousness, gregariousness and all the rest, we have at our best but a collection of half-truths. And half-truths can as conveniently be called half-untruths. None of us can take Adam's fall with that horror with which it is supposed to be taken. On the contrary, every reader's heart warms, like Dr. Tillyard's, with sympathy at

79. Perhaps the small syntactical crux in i, 26, may be mentioned here. Apparently the line is often taken to mean 'and justify the ways of God-to-man'. Newton certainly took it that way, cf. Waldock, *op. cit.*, p. 136, note 1. But I confess I cannot follow Professor Waldock's argument from viii. 224–6. 'To man' is not the same as 'with man'. Nor am I certain that his interpretation of these lines is the right one. Cf. also *Treatise*, Bk. I, Chap. 9. Col. ed., vol. xv, p. 98. What seems to be more decisive is that out of a hundred readers, ninety-nine will read 'and justify the-ways-of-God, to men'. And this, I suppose, not only because Milton's purpose rests on the two assumptions that (*a*) God's ways are just, and (*b*) that man can understand their justness, but mainly because this reading is also suggested by the music and cadence of the verse. But as this 'appeal to the ear' is easily brushed aside, I prefer to quote ll. 293–4 from *S.A.*, which settle this point once and for all:

> . . . *Just are the ways of God*
> *And justifiable to Men.*

80. *Op. cit.*, p. 96.

81. 'The Paradox of the Fall in Paradise Lost', *M.L.N.*, liii (Dec. 1938), 563–4.

Adam's sacrificial love. Even Mr. Lewis and Mr. Williams feel compelled to admit the 'half-nobility' of Adam, and regret that they cannot condone it. What cannot be stressed often enough is that Eve does not tempt or seduce Adam in the proper sense of the word. No doubt she tries to persuade Adam to taste the forbidden fruit,[82] but this attempt is not elaborated and lacks Milton's habitual fire. There is not the slightest hint of Eve using her 'female charms'[83] (this too is one of Milton's slanderous additions) to coax Adam into sinning. On the contrary, when the pinch comes, she too would rather renounce Deitie for her husband.[84] But the real Milton bursts forth with all his sweeping power as soon as Eve has finished her story.[85] This is a spontaneous and elementary outbreak of passion. It is love pure and undefiled at a really tragic level. Adam's eruption is volcanic and sudden:

> *. . . for with thee*
> *Certain my resolution is to Die;*
> *How can I live without thee, . . .*
>
> *P.L.* ix. 906–8
>
> *Should God create another* Eve, *and I*
> *Another Rib afford, yet loss of thee*
> *Would never from my heart.*
>
> *Ibid.* 911–13

To talk here with C. S. Lewis and Milton himself[86] of uxoriousness is almost as ridiculous as M. Saurat's 'chivalry'.[87] Here Addison is still the better guide when he said that we could all recognize our own human nature in Adam's weakness. 'It was the excess of love for Eve which ruin'd Adam and his posterity.' It goes without saying that Addison hastens to add at once 'that the author is justifyd in this particular by many of the fathers and the most orthodox writers'.

Addison reminds one of Miss Harriett Byron's opinion about Adam,[88] and Professor Waldock has indeed pitched on this delightful piece of Richardsonian day-dreaming to reproach Mr. Lewis with wishing that Adam had been not Adam, but Sir Charles Grandison.[89] What does not occur to Professor Waldock is to ask whether Milton may not in fact have desired us to entertain that wish. Milton's pious readers certainly did! After all, Sir Charles Grandison too managed to be Sir Charles Grandison, and this to the great admiration of Miss Byron and all the other parties concerned, last but not least Richardson

82. *P.L.* ix. 877–85.
83. Cf. also *P.R.* ii. 134.
84. *P.L.* ix. 884–5.
85. *P.L.* ix. 888–94, 896–901, 904–16.
86. *Treatise*, Bk. I, Chap. 11. Col. ed., vol. xv, p. 182.
87. *Op. cit.*, p. 169.
88. *Sir Charles Grandison*, (5th ed., 1766), v. 207.
89. Waldock, *op. cit.*, p. 53.

himself. We should beware of imputing our unregenerate twentieth-century feelings to Milton and his readers!

Of course the technical possibilities and requirements of the poem, put a heavy strain on it and are partly responsible for this split. God for instance, according to Professor Raleigh, is a 'whimsical tyrant', thereby putting Satan at an advantage. According to Professor Wilson Knight he is 'an even more verbose and intolerable person than Shakespeare's Caesar'.[90] Satan's hit, *Paradise Regained*, iii. 109–20, is a brilliant anticipation of H. G. Wells' 'venerable old man with an inordinate lust for propitiation and praise' and is only insufficiently countered by Jesus' answer (*ibid.*, ll. 121 ff.). Could God have been different? No, thought the late Archbishop Temple,[91] 'because an omnipotent protagonist is inevitably a bully'. Possibly yes, thinks Professor Grierson,[92] if Milton had been capable of reading the Hebrew prophets in another light. To this might be added a multitude of other difficulties, imposed indeed by the theme, but imposed by it *on Milton*. Some of them have already been seized upon by Johnson, others are continually discovered. To pick out a few random examples: Christ's foreknowledge of his triumph detracting from his sacrifice, God holding his enemies in derision and yet feeling necessarily 'endangered', Raphael is sent to guard the gates of hell during Creation against possible eruptions from hell,[93] assuring us in the same breath that God's omnipotent will alone might have prevented them.[94] The motivation which follows only helps to increase our uneasiness. Gabriel's regiment mounts guard in Paradise, whilst God foresees and permits Satan to erupt from hell.[95] In fairness to Gabriel it must be added that indeed he threatens that 'next time' (!)

Back to th'infernal pit I drag thee chaind,
And Seale thee so, as henceforth not to scorne
The facil gates of hell too slightly barred.

P.L. iv. 965–7

When Satan is caught, and about to fight it out with Gabriel, God intervenes with his golden scales, presumably with the sole purpose of enabling Satan to clear out in time to save his skin, and to be ready to attempt man's fall a second time with better success.[96] To put the lid on it all the guardian angels are solemnly acquitted.[97] The

90. *Op. cit.*, p. 133.
91. William Temple, *The Genius of English Poetry* (1939), p. 8.
92. *Op. cit.*, pp. 105, 110.
93. *P.L.* viii. 229–36.
94. *P.L.* viii. 237 ff.
95. *P.L.* iii. 80 ff.
96. *P.L.* iv. 996 ff.
97. *P.L.* x. 34 ff.

> *. . . many signes of power and rule*
> *Conferrd upon us, and Dominion giv'n*
> *Over all other Creatures*
>
> *P.L.* iv. 429–31

of which Adam boasts, are rather meagre and tame, consisting, as they do, mainly of the privilege to praise the Lord

> *. . . and extoll*
> *His bountie, following our delightful task*
> *To prune these growing Plants, and tend these Flours.*
>
> *Ibid.* 436–8

This idyllic setting for 'domestick Adam', not much different from the revivalist heaven, is a poor foil for the activity of hell. One is reminded of Mr. Lewis' beautiful comment on Spenser's contrast of the Garden of Adonis with the Bower of Acrasia. Mr. Lewis points out[98] that the characteristic of the Bower is enervation and lack of activity. 'There is not a kiss or an embrace in the island: only male prurience and female provocation.' Though Milton leaves us no doubt that kisses and embraces, to say the least, do take place in Paradise, yet compared with the teeming life of hell it cannot but strike us as another Bower of Acrasia.[99] Another striking illustration is provided by a comparison of the imagery used by Milton for his various protagonists.[100] One really gets the impression that Milton treated the heavenly party in a very stepmotherly way. The many inconsistencies between Milton's manner of presentation and commentary have already been noted.

In this connection I would also draw attention to the various oriental epithets of splendour and magnificence, applied by Milton to Satan. Mr. Rajan warns us not to be deceived by the exotic glamour of these words. To the seventeenth-century reader they conveyed less glamour and more hostility. The point has already been made by Newton in connection with i. 348, 'thir great Sultan' and x. 457, 'thir dark Divan', the latter evidently requiring the same response as 'conclave' in i. 795. But this undeniable undertone of negation should not blind us to the equally undeniable fascination of exotic words and settings. Certainly Milton is not Byron, but such words as 'orient gems',[101] already in use before Milton, show that more than pagan horror is involved. But Milton expressly goes out of his way to show that word-

98. C. S. Lewis, *The Allegory of Love* (1936), p. 332.
99. Cf. Chap. 4, and Tillyard, *op. cit.*, p. 282.
100. See Appendix B.
101. *P.L.* iii. 507 and iv. 238. Cf. the notes of Newton, Todd and Mitford.

music matters to him more than anything else. Even such important distinctions as 'Baptiz'd and Infidel',[102] fade away when he wants to riot with Aspramont, Montalban, Damasco, Trebisond, and the rest. A similar point can be made about the fallen angels' musical activities. As Milton could not yet know the *Screwtape Letters* which inform us that music is taboo in hell, he had to rely on Heywood.[103] But why had the infernal music to be in the '*Dorian* Mood',[104] the most grave and majestic of all? Already Newton noted that in his prose Milton uses Doric and grave as synonymous!

Some of these splits and incompatibilities Milton was obviously unable to see. Partly for lack of experience, mainly because, in the words of Professor Saurat, his fable was God's own truth. But all these explanations are insufficient. Milton was not as blind as that, and he has given ample proof of his freedom with regard to any fable or Biblical myth. When God's own fable was flexible enough, the various incidents and elaborations, which were of his own invention, are certainly not due to any constraint!

It would be futile to speculate how else Milton might or should have written his epic. That the theme *can* be treated differently, provided the poet is of a different temperament, has been shown by Vondel.[105] Vondel too, was a sincere and devout Christian, yet in many things Milton's exact opposite.[106] Vondel, like some subsequent poets, was 'a royalist in politics and a catholic in religion', whereas Milton was the defender of regicide[107] and opposed to Church government of any sort. Vondel's dramas too suffer from many shortcomings, inherent in himself and in his themes. But—and this is the important thing—his shortcomings are different from Milton's. For can we be so absolutely sure that Milton's was that standard seventeenth-century mind?

102. *P.L.* i. 582 ff.

103. Thomas Heywood: *The Hierarchie of the Blessed Angels* (London, 1635). 'The Fall of Lucifer', pp. 144 ff.

104. *P.L.* i. 550.

105. *Lucifer* (1654), *Adam in Ballingschap* (1664). Vondel's name is usually mentioned in connection with Milton's possible 'sources'. Cf. G. Edmundson: *Milton and Vondel, A Curiosity of Literature* (1885). A. Müller: *Ueber Milton's Abhängigkeit von Vondel* (1891). J. J. Moolhuizen: *Vondels Lucifer en Milton's Verloren Paradijs* (1895), and particularly Masson in *The Poetical Works of Milton* (1890), ii, 145–64. The main interest seems to me, however, to lie in the profound differences of spirit and conception, separating the two poets in spite of their many similarities.

106. Cf. Sir H. Grierson, art. 'Vondel' in *Hasting's Encyclopaedia of Religion and Ethics*, xii (1921), 637–40.

107. But cf. C. S. Lewis' excellent chapter 'Hierarchy'. Nevertheless the difference between Milton's version of hierarchy and obedience, and that of Vondel, as expressed in his dedication to Ferdinand III of his *Lucifer*, is significant.

Without making him M. Saurat's formidable Cabbalist, Milton, with all his Puritanism, was a very deep water under a deceptive surface. We can only gauge his depth and complexity when we compare him with the single-mindedness and transparency of such seventeenth-century types as Vondel and Bunyan.

As far as the seventeenth-century reader is concerned, I would suggest that the same thing happened with Milton's Satan as happened with his orthodoxy in general. Occasionally voices went up, suspecting his orthodoxy. In fact, the very suspicion already is a sort of condemnation. But Addison, and even Dr. Johnson, came out for the doctrinal purity of *Paradise Lost*; Bishop Newton declared: 'Let not the infidel glory', and distrusting his own judgement in this matter, referred to a more competent heresy-hunter, 'the learned Dr. Trapp', who too had found the poem *omni ex parte orthodoxorum*. After the publication of the *Treatise* it was of course easy to be wise and to re-read *Paradise Lost* in a new light, making manifest all things hidden.[108] To-day we are again less extreme, and we know that even if the heresies of the *Treatise* are not contradicted by *Paradise Lost*, they are neither necessarily implied or presupposed by it.[109] I think one must subscribe to Mr. Rajan's thesis, as long as it *only* means that *Paradise Lost can* be read and makes sense without the *Treatise*. But if it is taken to imply that the *Treatise* is irrelevant for a deeper and more complete understanding of the verse and its emotional and intellectual contents, then we must dissent. All we can say is that there *is* something in the poem which Milton's contemporaries did or could not suspect, but which *we* can read not only between but even in its very lines. Satan's case, I believe, is similar. It is impossible honestly to uphold that Satan is a satisfactory unity. But the duality in his presentation would have escaped the seventeenth-century reader on account of his strong presumptions on the subject, even as Bishop Newton's presumptions concerning the Trinity caused him to notice that the Son was described as

Equal to God, and equally enjoying
God-like fruition

iii. 306–7

simply overlooking the following lines, particularly l. 309

By Merit more then Birthright Son of God.

With a view to the patent duality in the presentation of Satan, and more generally, the split running through the whole poem, it seems

108. For an account of the shock the *Treatise* occasioned in theological circles, see H. McLachlan: *The Religious Opinions of Milton, Locke, and Newton*, (1941), pp. 23 ff.

109. Rajan, *op. cit.*, pp. 22–3, 35–6.

more reasonable to assume that all this was accepted without protest, because the seventeenth-century reader, under the influence of his spiritual climate, really saw the Satan Milton *intended* to write, sharing Milton's own ignorance as to what he actually had written. With the lapse of time, and with the greater mental distance gained towards the poem's theme, it could be viewed at closer quarters, and approached with a receptivity to some of its elements which had been clamped down by traditional religious presumptions. We can see *Paradise Lost*, as it were, enlarged; and in enlargements splits can appear as gulfs. What is a tiny speck or scratch on a film roll, becomes, when projected on to the screen, a great blur or stripe. But the blur and the stripe could not be there if the speck or scratch had not existed before.

To sum up: A fatal split in the presentation of Satan is undeniable. This split is inherent in the very texture of the verse, and is not due to our projecting something into the poem. The effect is that 'No remarks of Milton to remind us that Satan remains Satan can destroy . . . [the] . . . deep and noble significances'.[110] Though 'the fallen angels incorporate many of Milton's obvious aversions . . . the surface meaning of *Paradise Lost* appears to suffer from the unnecessary grandeur of Satan'.[111] The question we thus have to ask, is not whether or why Milton was a Satanist. If Blake thought that Milton was of the devil's party without knowing it, M. Saurat, though praising this passage as sheer genius, yet very aptly adds that Milton also was on God's side *and that he knew it*. The question rather is: How does it come about that Satan remains great in spite of all valiant attempts at degrading him? What are the sources of strength on which Satan draws? Why is Milton, not the Satanist, but the Puritan and Christian Soldier, *unable* to make his Satan as reprehensible as he knows that in fact he is? And why does Mr. Hamilton believe that 'there was room in Milton's heaven for a wholly splendid rebel'? He affirms the possibility of a Promethean rebellion, but does not say why. Why, in short, is the lesson to be drawn from the contrast hell-heaven 'spoilt and confused in the telling'?[112]

It is the answer to these questions which will be the object of the following chapters.

110. Wilson Knight, *op. cit.*, p. 134.
111. *Ibid.*, p. 126. 112. Hamilton, *op. cit.*, pp. 37, 41.

Chapter Two

PRIDE AND WORSE AMBITION

THE previous chapter, being a summary exposition of the present state of *Paradise Lost* criticism, has ostensibly tried to base itself on the text and to remain strictly within the bounds of literary criticism. But at the same time it also invited us, as it were, to overstep these boundaries. Literary criticism alone will frequently be found to be unable to answer the problems which it has raised. The points of cleavage shown to exist in Milton's poem, together form a *line* of cleavage which indicates the direction in which we should transcend it. What follows will consequently go to a large extent beyond the poem, wandering in strange fields, and a justification of this procedure may perhaps be pertinent here.

A perfect, or at least successful work of art, rests in itself. It has no umbilical cord binding it to its author; and for its understanding no data are needed besides those which it furnishes itself. Biographical, sociological, and historical facts may throw light on certain questions, correct minor points, even give new perspectives to the whole, but will never reveal any essential meanings. *Faust* is significant even without Goethe-biography, and one can read Shakespeare's Sonnets without having to pry into his bedroom. But to the extent that a great work of art is a failure, this method breaks down; the work is no longer self-sufficient. I am not speaking, of course, of cases where the failure is due to artistic insufficiency, for in that case there is no further problem. It is just a bad work of art, doomed to oblivion in due course. What interests us here is the undoubtedly good work of art which nevertheless reveals defects so fundamental as to justify an inquiry into the extra-artistic sources of its failure.

I consider *Paradise Lost* to be such a work of art. A great poem, if not one of the greatest, which has rightly commanded attention and admiration in the past, and which will probably continue to do so long after the rarefied subtleties of its critics, ancient and modern, have been forgotten. But at the same time one cannot but call it a failure. It has never fulfilled its self-avowed purpose, and will do so in an ever-decreasing measure, unless a gigantic 'conversion' throws us back a few centuries. *Paradise Lost* is full of unrelieved discord and unhealed splits, which are neither accidental nor extrinsic to the poetic quality of the verse. On the contrary, they are part of its texture and inherent in the very theme, or at least in the poet Milton when confronted with that very theme. It is therefore imperative to look for the springs of both Milton's strength and his failure, and I propose to do so not by continuing the analytical study of the text, though I shall repeatedly return to it, but by pitching on certain ideas and motives which seem to me to be at the nerve-centre of our problem. The choice of these is admittedly capricious and by no means exhaustive, and I am fully aware that I am laying myself open to the charge of stringing together a random choice of unconnected and disparate subjects. But as they all issue in what seems to me the central Miltonic problem, I would ask the reader to suspend judgement until this 'order in disorder' and the convergence on one point become clearer. My present purpose is strictly limited: to analyse these seemingly vital themes, to expound their meaning, to follow them in Milton's poetry, and to link them to the problem of the strength and failure of his epic. Some of these themes have been named and discussed in the preceding chapter. Another, and one of the most important, is that of Pride, the Greek 'original sin' of *hubris*.

As has already been remarked, there is no psychology of the fall in the sense of an objective account of the genesis of sin in the various protagonists of the fall-story. But such a psychology is both possible and significant if taken phenomenologically as the account of the fall-image in the human *psyche*. And this brings us to *hubris* as an eminently basic human problem, expressed in many of the most 'primordial images'. We find it as an almost ever-present nightmare in Greek culture, and as *the* interpretation of the Biblical fall-myth, gaining ground since apocryphal times, and becoming classic since Augustine and Gregory. It is obvious that Milton, whose egotism has proved a welcome target for the scarcely less arrogant irony of his biographers and critics,[1] should be strongly susceptible to this psychic and (in the language of myth) cosmic factor. No wonder that Satan has been considered as mirroring Milton's own vice. Certainly the force sustaining Satan and great part of the action of *Paradise Lost* is his tremendous and

1. 'The very centre of Milton's personality seems . . . to consist in a powerful feeling of egotism and pride, in the fullest self-consciousness of a tremendous personality'. Saurat, *op. cit.*, p. xv. Cf. also the quotation from Johnson, p. 38.

unbounded pride. The Mount Niphates speech is actually a monologue on the *hubris* theme.

What precisely does *hubris* mean, and how does it link up with Biblical and Christian thought? *Hubris*, the Greek word for pride, seems to be the characteristic of Greek culture[2] and its dominating problem. It is an aspect of what Bertrand Russell[3] calls the Greek 'theory or feeling about the Universe', and as Greece is the mainspring of western civilization, it is of extreme importance to us. After all, the problems of the Greek world, and the largely different ones of Jewish and Biblical thought, are part of our own world and essential to an understanding of the Graeco-Jewish dialectics both within Christianity and within western civilization.

Hubris can be defined as the 'personification of overweening pride in which man, heedless of his mortal nature and losing all sense of measure, allows his skill, his power and his good fortune to make him arrogant towards gods and men, thus bringing down upon himself the avenging punishment of the gods, *Nemesis*'.[4] Observe that this definition might almost be taken from a description of Satan's fall. As a symptom of human self-assertion and progressing individuation, *hubris* is a problem of consciousness and thus belongs to the problems attending the growth of the human mind. It is no accident that we find so much care of *hubris* in Greece, the country which has bequeathed to us philosophy and science. If the Greeks did not develop the technical sciences it was precisely their fear of *hubris* which, according to Bertrand Russell, prevented them from doing so. In fact, the idea that Pride was not only at the origin of the fall, but also of science, has long been a commonplace:

Pride then was not, nor arts that pride to aid
Man walked with beast joint-tenant of the shade

. . . . .

2. If taken absolutely this is, of course, a gross and unwarranted overstatement. One should not dogmatize about racial differences, and most human problems and symbols are found everywhere, though in different forms. *Hubris* occurs in the Bible (Tower of Babel) and in the Babylonian Etana and Gilgamesh stories. Nevertheless different races and cultures seem to develop certain characteristics and psychic forces more than others, constellating thereby peculiar psychic possibilities, which manifest themselves in typical patterns of conscious and unconscious creative expression. It is interesting to note Professor van der Leeuw disclaiming *hubris* as a Greek peculiarity (*La Religion dans son essence et ses manifestations: Phénoménologie de la Religion* (1948), p. 308) only to admit later (p. 459) that it was 'the great sin' for the Greeks 'who could never abstain from it'.

3. *History of Western Philosophy* (1946), p. 134.

4. Roscher, *Lexicon der Griech. und Röm. Mythologie*, i, 2, 2767–8.

PRIDE AND WORSE AMBITION

Pride still is aiming at the blest abodes,
Men would be angels, angels would be gods.

(Pope, *Essay on Man*, i. 173 ff.)

Similarly Rousseau could declare: *Toutes les sciences, et la morale même, sont nées de l'orgueil humain*, and Montaigne (*Apologie de Raymond Sebond*): *Le soing de s'augmenter en sagesse et en science, ce feut la première ruyne du genre humain; . . . l'orgueil est sa perte et sa corruption.* This provides, as we shall presently see, the setting for the Miltonic condemnation of civilization.[5] As an interesting sidelight I would quote from the Dutch thinker Fokke Sierksma's criticism of Sartre: 'The absolutist western rationalism has . . . taken over, together with the Greek reason, also the Greek sin: *hubris.*' This formulation contains more truth than is suspected at first sight; pride and the development of self-conscious intellect belong together.

The archetypal imagery for the emergence of consciousness is varied and rich in symbolism. It is usually based on that of the emergence of individual life, whilst the supposed cosmic reference of the latter is really indicative of unconscious processes. Thus the mother-image stands for: the womb out of which things are born, the primordial chaos out of which the world emerges,[6] the great deep, the amorphous matter out of which structure, differentiated existence and organic, i.e., organized life are produced. Actually all these are symbols of consciousness emerging from the womb of the unconscious: a painful and protracted birth-process. But parallel to this upward drive, there is a strong reactionary tendency of inertia, a force resisting the impulsion towards higher differentiation, a sort of psychic gravitation tending back to the lowest point. It is, in other words, a wish to return to the womb, that is to say to chaos. As long as this urge is still alive, chaos (or the womb-image) represents a potential danger, and stimulates the appropriate reactions for self-preservation, in this case: *hubris.*

Woman, particularly in her role as mother, but also because touching man's instinctive, natural and most uncontrollable part, is thus not only symbolical of the birth-giving, feeding and protecting, but also of the dark, irrational and threatening side of the world and of our own unconscious.[7] Certainly in a civilization determined by man, the mother, i.e., female image, can be expressive of negative emotions. But whatever the attitude toward's one's origins and destiny, growth means from somewhere. It implies that one's roots are in the earth and not in the

5. Cf. pp. 81 ff.

6. The Babylonian *tiamat*, still traceable in the *tehom* (abyss) of *Gen.* i. 2, belongs to the same group of images.

7. Cf. the incident of Faust's descent to the 'mothers' in Pt. II of Goethe's *Faust.*

air. The panicky fear-reaction to the threat of one's origin[8] can lead to an extreme separation which, because impossible, must needs end in disaster.[9]

Grossly and schematically speaking we might say that the human *psyche*, confronted with its fate (or calling) is beset by two principal temptations. The one is to avoid progress and to try to undo one's birth. It is the attempt to return into the womb. The other is the typical fear response: a panicky rush towards new heights, lest one be submerged again. It is the attempt to sever oneself completely from one's mother. The one seeks liberation from the agony of new responsibilities by remaining within the vicious circle of natural life, and living with the rhythm of nature, the alternation of 'birth copulation and death, birth, copulation and death', of work and ecstasy of senses. This is the basis of nature cults, the worship of Baäl to which Israel was ever prone to return. The other hopes to evade this temptation by soaring too high unto the light, leaving all that is irrational, instinctive, and natural far behind.

The latter is the Greek situation. The liberation from the original Creto-Mycaenian matriarchal system, and the ascendancy of the male symbol[10] are expressions of a tremendous psychic impetus which, in fact, proved of far-reaching and decisive importance. But this movement is still obsessed by the fear of the origins which it has overcome and transcended. It is accompanied by a bad conscience of its own: the fear of going too far, of soaring too high, of substituting a reckless selfishness for the process of legitimate individuation. Thence the

8. Cf. C. G. Jung, *Wandlungen u. Symbole der Libido* (3rd ed., 1938), passim (index), and 'Psychologische Aspekte des Mutterarchetypus' in *Eranos-Jahrbuch* (1938), p. 412 on the symbol of the *mater devorans*. Appropriately enough, the Bible not only enjoins that man should cleave unto his wife and be one flesh with her, but also that he first '*leave* his father and mother'. (*Gen.* ii. 24.)

9. For the indispensable *tiefenpsychologische* background of what is only superficially indicated in these and the following paragraphs, see e.g., E. Neumann *Ursprungsgeschichte des Bewusstseins* (1949), his analysis of the Uroboros, as well as his account of the various stages of incest with and severance from the parents, and in particular of the various levels of parent images (such as the 'higher' and 'lower' father and mother image).

10. I am stating here a possibility, fully aware that it is no more than one of the many doubtful hypotheses concerning Greek origins. Although it is presumptuous for a layman to rush in where scholars fear to tread, I have simply chosen that version which tallies best with the system of psychology which I have adopted. I do not believe that the present argument would be seriously affected if the facts concerning this particular point were different. For the question as such see Charles Piccard, *Les Religions Préhelléniques* (1948), pp. 80–3, and his chapter 'La Religion Continentale à L'Epoque Mycénienne' and the bibliography given there. See also Harrison, *Themis*, Chap. 11.

significance of such *hubris* legends as of Icarus, Phaeton, Bellerophon and others[11] which are all reduceable to one fundamental awareness: Don't aspire too high; the higher you soar, the surer you are to fall. Milton has clearly stated this old lesson

> *. . . who aspires must down as low*
> *as high he soard.*
>
> *P.L.* ix. 169–70

The Greek spirit aspires too high, seeking the idea and spurning the *materia*. Appropriately enough, Parmenides' philosophical poem begins with a Phaeton-like ascent.[12] We shall see in due course how acute this *hubris*-problem was with Milton, and in how far it supplies a key to many of the difficulties raised by his poems.

The other possibility is illustrated by the Jewish experience. The fundamental danger, as presented in the books of the Old Testament, is not that of aspiring too high, but of not aspiring high enough, i.e., of infidelity to a spiritual calling by harking back to the eternal rhythm of nature: 'Let us serve the Baälim.' But they were fighting a hopeless battle against a God who would not let them sink back to the level of existence from which he had called them of all the families of the earth to a destiny of their own. 'So the Lord alone did lead him, and there was no strange God with him.'[13] Underlying this idea of chosenness was a sense of fate, of the inevitability of God's ways, of the threat that 'I, the Lord, thy God am a jealous God'.[14] When the Old Testament period of Jewish history draws towards a close, the men and women of Judah could say to Jeremiah:

'As for the word that thou hast spoken unto us in the name of the Lord, we will not hearken unto thee. But we will certainly do whatsoever thing goeth forth out of our own mouth, to burn incense unto the queen of heaven, and to pour out drink offerings unto her, as we have done, we, and our fathers, our kings, and our princes, in the cities of Judah, and in the streets of Jerusalem: for then had we plenty of victuals, and were well, and saw no evil.'[15]

But the prophet could answer them:

'Because ye have burned incense, and because ye have sinned against the Lord and have not obeyed the voice of the Lord, nor walked in his law, nor in his statutes, nor in his testimonies, therefore this evil is happened unto you as at this day. . . . Behold, I will watch over them

11. Which Milton has not failed duly to mention, *P.L.* iii. 466 ff.

12. Diels, *Fragmente der Vorsokratiker* (3rd ed., 1912), i. 148 ff. particularly ll. 1–12.

13. *Deut.* xxxii. 12. 14. *Exod.* xx. 5. 15. *Jer.* xliv. 16–17.

for evil, and not for good: and all the men of Judah that are in the land of Egypt shall be consumed by the sword and by the famine, until there be an end of them.'[16]

The same is the message of Ezekiel's devastating vision.[17] The prophets were the men whose task it was to keep alive the consciousness of an ineluctable chosenness for a higher calling. They knew that God had them by the neck, pulling them up with violent shakes, whenever they tried to fall back into the norms and forms 'of the nations'. The peculiar sin of *hubris* simply had no place here, because the aspiration towards heaven was experienced and symbolized not as an urge from below, but as a calling and irresistible pull from above. They were *called* by God, therefore the great sin was to stray after the gods of the earth and to burn incense to the *queen* of heaven.[18] On the other hand they always remained so deeply rooted in the earth, that the danger of a disincarnate spirituality never came into prominence until the end of the Old Testament period. Neither the belief in a soul as distinct from the body and immortal, nor philosophic idealism, originated in Biblical Judaism.

In glaring contrast to this experience stands the manner of achievement of Greek emancipation to consciousness. Here the urge of progress is an inner dynamism. It is therefore liable to go too far and to be haunted by a sense of wrongdoing. Necessary and understandable as this flight to heaven may be, it is accompanied by the unconscious knowledge that man's place is earth. Greek spirituality aspires to transcend this earth, and knows it must fall again. The Jew is called by his God, but tries to live with Baäl, and his prophet has to tell him:

'And that which cometh into your mind shall not be at all, that ye say We will be as the heathen, as the families of the countries, to serve wood and stone. As I live, saith the Lord God, *surely with a mighty hand, and with a stretched out arm and with fury poured out, will I rule over you.*'[19]

16. *Ibid.* 23, 27.

17. *Ezek.* viii. 7–18.

18. Indeed, the measure of *hubris*-fear can be decisive for the development of religious ideas. In a *hubris*-possessed culture, man's equality with God can only be viewed with horror and recoiling. As Miss Harrison has put it (*Themis*, p. 468) '. . . there grew up the disastrous notion that between god and man there was a great gulf fixed, that communion was no more possible. To attempt to pass this gulf was *hubris*, it was *the* sin against the gods.' In the comparatively *hubris*-free Biblical world the idea could be born of man as called to an *imitatio Dei*: 'Be ye holy, even as your father which is in heaven is holy'. But cf. the highly interesting quotation from Plutarch in Harrison's *Themis*, p. 80, as also the quotation from Montaigne, p. 43.

19. *Ezek.* xx. 32–3. This difference between Biblical and Greek *prise de conscience* can hardly be overrated from a phenomenological point of view. Forms of religion and culture greatly depend on whether one approaches God by building the Tower of

The above sheds an interesting light on the background of the fall-myth and on the various psychic constellations out of which it could develop. For whereas in Biblical myths 'sin' is frequently connected with woman, as representing man's danger-zone: the unconscious (Eve gives the forbidden fruit to Adam; Job's wife is the unwitting partner of Satan by bidding her husband to 'curse God and die'), the sin of *hubris* can, by way of figure of speech, be called the hypertrophy of masculinity—at least in so far as the growth of individuality and self-consciousness is comprehended under the male symbol. It is just possible that the homosexuality[20] of Greek culture, as well as its contempt for woman are one aspect of that particular spirituality which also succeeded in inventing idealism.

If we take the castration symbol as meaning cessation of personality and individuality in its progressive and fertile sense, then the inevitable result of hybridic inflation is the 'higher' or 'patriarchal' castration. To be hurled down from heaven into the underworld is only one of the many images for this 'annihilation by the Spirit'. At the other end of the scale stands the 'lower' or 'matriarchal' castration, the annihilation by the earth-mother. The result is in both cases the same, as ultimately

---

Babel, or because: '. . . the Lord hath taken you, and brought you forth out of the iron furnace, even out of Egypt, to be unto him a people of inheritance. . . . For ask now of the days that are passed, which were before thee, since the day that God created man upon the earth, and ask from the one side of heaven unto the other, whether there hath been any such thing as this great thing is, or hath been heard like it? Did ever people hear the voice of God speaking out of the midst of the fire, and live? Or hath God assayed to go and take him a nation from the midst of another nation, by temptations, by signs, and by wonders, and by war, and by a mighty hand, and by a stretched out arm, and by great terrors, according to all that the Lord your God did for you in Egypt before your eyes?' (*Deut.* iv. 20, 32–4.) Only thus too is it possible to grasp the full depth of difference between the Greek *eros* and the Christian *agape*. Cf. van der Leeuw, *op. cit.*, pp. 501–2, and the references given there in the notes.

20. As a rule, however, homosexuality is a symptom of subjection to the 'mother'. As a social phenomenon it appears where a primitive male society begins to crystallize as the initial stage of what is to develop later into the state. I would mention in this connection a story about a tribe of South American Indians, which is too good to be omitted, as it illustrates the connection between *hubris* as an upward movement symbolizing the emergence of a higher and more individuated consciousness, and homosexuality as an expression of the urge for independence from the female principle. In this matriarchal tribe the men are wont to 'emancipate' themselves at regular seasons by sitting on the roofs of their huts, indulging in homosexual practices, and singing: 'We are we.' When after some time nature asserts her superior strength in the form of hunger, these Indian Phaethons have to climb down again and resume their normal life. I am indebted to Miss Marie-Louise von Franz for this story, although, unfortunately, I cannot trace it at present.

it matters little whether one loses reality (which implies heaven *and* earth) and one's self through a heavenly father or through the *magna mater*. The only way of life is the middle way—though not Aristotle's, but that of Buddha: 'between pest and cholera'. But apparently Greek and Jew must approach this golden mean from the different sides of it on which they find themselves. *Piety* is the supreme virtue of the hero. In the awe and reverence he bears to the gods he recognizes his limitations and thus safeguards his self. The supreme symbol of the Jew is circumcision.[21] As a memento aiming at the limitation of sensuality, it is at the same time the consciousness of being called by God, sealed in the flesh. The Biblical account represents the institution of the rite as the final touch to God's covenant with Abraham, and it is as the 'covenant of Abraham' that circumcision still functions to-day in Jewish rite and liturgy.

It is fairly obvious that Christianity has lined up with the 'heaven' cultures. In spite of valiant attempts to effect a synthesis with the earth, and actually conceiving of the beginning of the Church as of the foundation of a kingdom, and although a higher relation to the mother-image was attained in the figure of the Holy Virgin, yet the essential hostility to, or at least estrangement from, the 'earth' and the body remained. Even the historical failure of the Church must to a very great extent be ascribed to her refusal or inability to tackle the more earthly problems, such as, e.g., the economic or the political power problem.[22] In fact, the great triumphs of Christian martyrdom and self-abnegation are not without their psychologically less reputable aspects, and the Gospel at least once clearly refers to the 'higher' castration-complex of a spirituality which does not succeed in liberating its anima, and which thus refuses creative fertility by becoming 'one flesh':

'For there are some eunuchs which were born so from their mother's womb: and there are some eunuchs, which were made eunuchs of men: and there are eunuchs, which have made themselves eunuchs for the kingdom of heaven's sake. He that is able to receive it, let him receive it.' (*Mat.* xix. 12.)

Consequently, when the primitive simplicity of the story of *Genesis* ii had to undergo later, apocryphal elaboration, something very interesting happened. Jewish legend pitched on the sensual aspect, whereas patristic speculation, at bottom the Greek mode of thought, concentrated on the *hubris* theme. This does not mean that the one motive was

21. The relation of circumcision to the castration problem is beautifully expressed in German *Be-schneiden* and *Ver-schneiden*.

22. John Hadham, *God and Human Progress* (1944), Chap. 5, and Tawney, *Religion and the Rise of Capitalism*, *passim*.

chosen in ignorance of the other. St. Augustine expressly recognizes two cardinal sins: *superbia* (*hubris*) and *concupiscentia* (sensuality). The interest of the case lies in the fact that of the two vices only one is really 'cardinal' for the psychic reality of Greek and Jew, and that each has projected his peculiar vice into his version of the fall-myth. It thus came about that out of two traditional and accepted possibilities, the one remained merely mentioned, whilst the other was given a central position. When later Jewish legend developed the idea of a fall of angels, the Old Testament Apocrypha loved to dwell on *Genesis* vi. 4, i.e., sensuality, in spite of the splendid *hubris* passage in *Isaiah* xiv. 12–15.[23] On the other hand the Fathers, though perfectly aware of the lure of female beauty, yet preferred to make pride the cornerstone of their theology of fall and sin. It is only in patristic literature that the fall becomes distinctly luciferic.[24]

The more material version of pride is the ambition to rule, 'to set oneself in glory above one's peers'. This ambition is a symbiotic relation to the world which intends to give the individual a sense of security by presenting him with a concrete focus for his individuality: he himself as set over and against the others, and disposing of them. Obviously the various forms of pride are as a rule not treated separately by moralists and poets, although the Church soon discovered that spiritual pride required some special attention as a particularly insidious vice.

The exact earthly counterpart, in Milton, of the fall in heaven, is not Adam's fall, but the episode told in Book XII, 24 ff. Nimrod's *hubris* preludes the best-known *hubris*-myth: the Tower of Babel.[25] Particularly ll. 36–7:

> *And from Rebellion shall derive his name,*
> *Though of Rebellion others he accuse*

which clearly refer to the monarchist claim in general and to Charles in particular, ring truly satanic, and have moreover the merit of clearly and explicity conveying Milton's attitude. For, as has already been repeatedly said, the occasions are rare where Milton succeeds in giving satisfactory utterance to his beliefs. More often the 'fair equalitie, fraternal state' is found in the satanic party, made up, it is true, of 'a crew whom like ambition joins', whereas God's is the 'Empire tyrranous', and heaven, as Professor Wilson Knight says, is a totalitarian state.

23. Milton wavers rather amusingly in his interpretation of the *Genesis* passage. Cf. *P.L.* xi. 621 ff. with *P.L.* v. 443–8 and *P.R.* ii. 178–81.

24. For a short but very informative account of the development of the ideas about Satan and the fall, see Langton, *op. cit.*, Chaps. 3–7.

25. *P.L.* xii. 41–5.

At first I thought that Liberty and Heav'n
To heav'nly souls had bin all one; but now
I see that most through sloth had rather serve,
Ministring Spirits, traind up in Feast and Song;
Such hast thou arm'd, the Ministrelsie of Heav'n
Servilitie with freedom to contend.

P.L. vi. 164–9

At any rate, the fact alone that hell often seems to be what heaven *ought* to have been, and that at times we find ourselves wondering whether certain descriptions refer to Charles or to Cromwell, sufficiently shows that Milton has not really solved his problems.

It goes without saying that Milton condemns both pride and ambition,[26] and so indeed does even Satan.[27] Hume comments:

'Pride is a kind of excessive and vicious self esteem, that raises men in their own opinions above what is just and right: but ambition is that which adds fuel to this flame . . . which makes our author stigmatize ambition as a worse sin than pride.'

And Pearce, quoted by Newton, says:

'Pride is the vice confined in itself . . . ambition the vice that carried him at being equal with God: and was not this vice the worst of the two? I observe that Satan always lays the blame on his ambition.'

Very characteristic too is Milton's formulation 'better to reign in hell than serve in heaven',[28] of which Newton notes: 'this is a wonderfully fine improvement upon Prometheus answer to Mercury in Aesch. Prom. Vinct . . ., it was a memorable saying of Julius Caesar . . . the reader will observe how properly the saying is here applied . . . a sentiment worthy of Satan, and of him only'. The opposite ideal of 'Fair Equality, fraternal state' is a community based on a hierarchy of genuine values, where as a consequence service takes on a different meaning; a meaning which Milton was not always very successful in conveying, and which is expressed very trenchantly and almost as a conscious repartee to Caesar by the Rabbis:[29] 'Be a tail to lions rather than a head to foxes.' The same sentiment, Milton's profoundest conviction, is stated on his behalf by Abdiel.[30]

Pride and ambition thus appear as an inordinate striving and trespass of one's bounds. This, in fact, is also the purport of the definition already quoted.[31] When looked at that way, it becomes clear

26. *P.L.* i. 36–44.
27. *P.L.* iv. 40.
28. *P.L.* i. 263.
29. *Aboth* iv.
30. *P.L.* vi. 172 ff. The best commentary to this speech I know of, is Mr. C. S. Lewis' chapter 'Hierarchy'.
31. See p. 29.

that this problem of knowing one's limits and keeping within them, is basically that of temperance: the problem of the right measure. Obviously, from the point of view of poetic expression and the emotive value of words, it does matter a good deal whether we define original sin as pride, disobedience or intemperance. Essentially, however, there is no objection to regarding intemperance as the right word, provided it is supplemented by its proper context and understood in its full significance. 'Inordinate' is therefore the adjective, used or understood, qualifying the various sins, which appear as so many guises, forms, and nuances of the temperance problem.

Both pride and sensuality find their place in this definition. We might therefore say that man's trespassing has shown itself as going into two directions, to wit pride and sensuality. The two are twins, belonging to all human experience, although the centre of gravity may shift from the one to the other in different cultures or circumstances. Corresponding therewith we have noted the traditional versions of the fall-myth. Its elaboration actually consisted in various combinations of the pride and sensuality motives, so that Milton could feel it not unbecoming his context to charge Satan with additional lust and incest, and to give to the forbidden fruit the effects of an aphrodisiac.

Milton is of exemplary significance, because with him both drifts are equally strong. He is an intensified mixture of Greek and Jew, of genuine New Testament Christianity and Old Testament Judaism. His life is largely dominated by his struggle against sensuality. Against his pride, I am afraid, he did not struggle at all; partly because he invariably so sublimated it that he could identify his aspirations with God, and partly because of his lack of self-knowledge which rendered him blind to his own stoic vice. This lack of self-criticism is amusingly illustrated by Milton's own words in his *Second Defence* concerning those who '. . . endeavour to throw off the yoke, not from the love of genuine liberty (which a good man only loves and knows how to obtain) but from the impulses of pride and little passions'. This is almost a literal anticipation of Johnson's stricture: 'Milton's republicanism was, I am afraid, founded in an envious hatred of greatness, and sullen desire of independence, in petulance impatient of control, and pride disdainful of superiority . . . he hated all whom he was required to obey . . . he felt not so much the love of liberty as repugnance to authority.' Probably it never occurred to Milton to view himself from this angle, so that Professor Hanford could rightly say that 'no student of the poet need to be told how impossible it is to separate his general opinions and purposes from his more intimate emotions, or his propagandist utterances from his dominant instinct for self-portraiture and self-justification'. Professor Grierson puts it thus: 'if he was moved by personal motives, they were always sublimated to take the aspect of high ideals',[32] and M. Saurat: 'because of his peculiar pride, his egotism will always need to be identified with something great . . . and Milton will end by identifying himself with God'.[33]

But there is more to it than that. That Satan's pride is at times not felt as reprehensible enough, whilst the Father's disdainful superiority in *Paradise Lost* is scarcely balanced by the Son's speeches, is bad enough. And of *Paradise Regained*, i. 201–4, Professor Saurat says:[34] 'The whole of the presentation of Christ in the first book is vitiated by intolerable self-consciousness.' Christ, in fact, betrays a typically stoic frame of mind. But his words in *Paradise Regained*, iii. 46 ff. are far worse. Here is pagan aristocracy speaking; the words might come from Shakespeare's Coriolanus. One understands why Archbishop Temple said: '*Paradise Lost* . . . is very bad drama. *Paradise Regained* is worse.'[35] Christ's words are quite in keeping with his role of a redeemer who calmly leaves the mass of men to 'Satan's perverted world', and whose heaven is peopled by the minority of heroes who managed to stay outside the herd.[36] We touch here the unchristian, i.e., Greek pole of Milton's mind, which Lord David Cecil[37] has so well described: 'He was a philosopher rather than a devotee. His imagination was lucid and concrete, unlit by heavenly gleams . . . nor was his moral sensibility a Christian one. The stoic virtues, fortitude, temperance, above all, moral independency, were what he valued. He did not live by faith, scorned hope, and was indisposed to charity, while pride, so far from being the vice which Christianity considers it, was to Milton the mark of a superior nature. . . . As an exposition of Christian belief *Paradise Lost* and *Paradise Regained* are failures.' Similarly Professor Grierson says: 'If *Paradise Lost* (and even *Paradise Regained*) seems to many people to-day imperfectly Christian in spirit, it is not because of any explicitly heretical doctrines . . . but because Milton's scale of values is not that of the orthodox and sincere Christian, Evangelical or Catholic'.[38] Already Raleigh had noted the ultimately non-religious basis on which Milton rests his universe, and, more biographically, Dr. Tillyard[39] has pointed out how Milton's stoical bent of mind was all he could fall back on after the Restoration disillusionment.

It is apposite here to examine briefly Milton's attitude to Stoicism.

32. *Cross-currents in English Literature of the Seventeenth Century* (1929), p. 237.
33. *Op. cit.*, p. 48. 34. *Ibid.*, p. 234. 35. *Op. cit.*, p. 8.
36. Grierson, *Milton and Wordsworth*, p. 81.
37. Introduction to *The Oxford Book of Christian Verse*, pp. xxi–xxii.
38. *Op. cit.*, pp. 99–100. 39. *Op. cit.*, p. 294.

The question is relevant not only in the light of the incisive but indisputable words of Lord Cecil, but chiefly because of the close relation discussed above between *hubris* and some aspects of Greek culture of which Stoicism is in many respects the purest and most extreme expression. The psychic constellation described earlier and of which Stoicism is an offshoot, is not foreign to Milton. M. Saurat may have overrated the role of sensuality and passion in Milton's life, but even so it was considerable enough. I do not intend here to assess the relative importance of the two cardinal vices, pride and sensuality, with Milton, but it is interesting to note how much scholars diverge in their evaluations, both biographically and also in interpreting *Paradise Lost*. Professor Saurat sees lust and passion as the essence of the fall.[40] His text is Book IX, 1008–45: the sensual crisis follows the eating of the fruit, and only thereafter comes the penitent knowledge of good and evil, rather in the style of *omne animal*, etc. Similarly Satan joins incest to rebellion, and Milton, in his poetic paraphrase of *James* i. 15, equates Satan with lust.[41] And again: 'Satan is not only pride. He

40. *Op. cit.*, p. 153.

41. *Ibid.*, p. 154. It may not be amiss to say here a few words about this incident and the great discoveries M. Saurat claims to have made in this connection. The incest symbolism in the *Zohar* has nothing to do with Milton's Allegory of Sin, the similarities being too external and fortuitous. Once Satan begets a daughter as Zeus did Athene, the incest situation is given for a poet who is determined to introduce this element—there being no other person, and in particular no divine mother with whom incest could be possible, in the Biblical (i.e., here Miltonic) heaven. Moreover, the father-daughter relationship of the *Zohar* is no 'incest' proper, but an inner-divine process of development. Foreign as the cabbalistic symbolism may be to Biblical imagery, it is nevertheless a fruit of the Biblical tree, because, in a way, Eve too is Adam's daughter: 'Woman, because she was taken out of man' (*Gen.* ii. 23). The Biblical creation-myth is conspicuous for having no 'mother', no womb out of which being arises, no *magna mater* as source of all things. Woman is created in the first place not as mother but as the wife of man. Only thereafter does she also become the 'mother of all living' (*Gen.* iii. 20). She is created as 'a help answering him' (lit.: opposite him, *Gen.* ii. 18) because 'it is not good that man should be alone', and the sense of marriage is precisely that man should '*leave* his father and mother, and cleave unto his wife: and they shall be one flesh' (*Gen.* ii. 24). Evidently this is the first and most beautiful statement of the animus-anima relation, possibly having arisen as a protest against the supremacy of the oriental mother-image from which Gilgamesh still tries to fight free. The *tehom* of *Gen.* i. 2, is a weak linguistic echo of the Babylonian *tiamat* and an adumbration of what the creation myth *might* have been. That means that for a Biblical unconscious, i.e., for the psychic structure and level represented by the Old Testament (though not by the *OT* alone), the mythological incest, when necessary, must be constellated as a father-daughter relationship, contrasting with the mother-son incest of most other myths. On the incest-mythology see Neumann, *op. cit.* The cabbalistic symbolism will be discussed in Dr. S. Hurwitz's forthcoming study: *Archetypische Motive in der Chassidischen Mystik*, part. his chapter

is passion in general. He is, in particular, sensuality—and Milton gratuitously put this upon him.'[42] But in the end he too has to admit that in the main Milton follows Augustine and that, in spite of *Paradise Lost*, v. 443–9 and *Enoch*, pride is the chief motive of the angels' fall.[43] On the other hand Dr. Tillyard contends that even Samson's failure was due first and foremost to pride, and only in the second place to sensuality.[44] According to him the analogy between Samson and Milton must be found chiefly in their wounded pride.[45] Both rave against women in the consciousness of having made fools of themselves. Professor Grierson's words about Samson are almost identical: Samson's is 'a very Miltonic repentance in which there is more of wounded pride than of Christian repentance which includes forgiveness'.[46] I think this consensus of opinion significant, particularly since no one denies the personal meaning of *Samson Agonistes*. Pride is Milton's most dominant characteristic, and without being able to prove anything, I must record my strong feeling that this is closely connected with his sensuality. He is moved by a Biblical affirmation of the material world, and at the same time by a Platonic idealism and positively stoic contempt for the passions and senses. This *élan* towards a heaven of Platonic ideas suggests the well-known hybridic escape from the dangers of this earth. It is true that Samson, Milton's nearest approach to a synthesis, easily overcomes Dalila's temptation, but only by (prudently) not giving her a chance. And his sudden outbreak of fury shows how great he felt the danger to be.

No doubt Milton believed in the flesh. As Dr. Tillyard says, he rather wanted to materialize the angels than to etherialize mankind.[47] His conscious and authentic Hebraism, the desire for unity between material reality and spiritual aspiration, pervades his philosophy, and also prompted his participation in the revolution. It caused him to differ from some of St. Augustine's 'crabb'd opinions', and made him

---

'Conjunctio-Mystik'. The best-known example is, of course, the birth of Jesus from the Virgin Mary. Our ears seem to catch the well-known mythological overtones in Dante's beautiful hymn (*Paradiso* xxxiii, 1–6):

Vergine madre, figlia del tuo figlio
umile ad alta più che creatura
termine fisso d'eterno consiglio

tu se' colei, che l'umana natura
nobilitasti sì che il suo Fattore
non disdegnò di farsi sua fattura.

42. *Ibid.*, p. 216. 43. *Ibid.*, p. 274.
44. *Op. cit.*, p. 337. See also *S.A.*, 522–34.
45. *Ibid.*, p. 346. 46. *Op. cit.*, p. 142. 47. *Op. cit.*, p. 383.

reject celibacy and extol marriage and sex-life. But at the same time Milton remains deeply distrustful. He senses the danger lurking behind Eve, Dalila and the story in *Genesis* vi. 4, and he is fully aware of the fatal ambivalence of the *Ewig-weibliche*. No wonder that he heartily concurs with St. Paul's teaching concerning the inferiority of women,[48] and proclaims as the burden of *Samson Agonistes* that

> . . . *Gods universal Law*
> *Gave to the man despotic power*
> *Over his female in due awe,*
> *Nor from that right to part an hour,*
> *Smile she or lowre.*

1053–7

His numerous outbursts against the other sex have provided many of his critics and biographers with cheap material for making fun. But it is this fear of being 'pulled down', and the consequently hostile reflex-attitude to nature, which links him with the Greek, and particularly with the stoic world. For Stoicism can be described as the final stage of *hubris*. Its ideal, the completely rational man, beyond the reach of all the irrational realities of this world, the philosopher, unmoved and unmovable, is really equal to God, because sufficient unto himself. It is as such that he is condemned by Milton:

> *The Stoic last in Philosophic pride,*
> *By him call'd vertue; and his vertuous man,*
> *Wise, perfect in himself, and all possessing*
> *Equal to God, oft shames not to prefer,*
> *As fearing God nor man, contemning all*
> *Wealth, pleasure, pain or torment, death and life,*
> *Which when he lists, he leaves, or boasts he can,*
>
> . . . . .
>
> *Alas what can they teach, and not mislead;*
> *Ignorant of themselves, of God much more,*
> *And how the world began, and how man fell*
> *Degraded by himself, on grace depending?*

P.R. iv. 300 ff.

and well described by Satan as

> *A mind not to be changed by Place or Time*

P.L. i. 253

48. *Treatise, de gubern. spec. hominis ante lapsum:* Woman inferior, 1 *Cor.* xi. 7–9. Power of husband increased after fall, *Gen.* iii. 6, 1 *Pet.* iii. 6, 1 *Tim.* ii. 12–14. (Col. ed., vol. xv, p. 121.)

The commentators are certainly right in referring this to Stoicism. 'These are some of the extravagances of the Stoics, and could not be better ridiculed than they are here by being put in the mouth of Satan in his present situation',[49] and 'This was a maxim of the Stoics, the most obstinate and uncompromising sect of all the old philosophers, who often carried it to a preposterous extent. It is here quite characteristic of the doggedness and vanity of Satan.'[50]

Stoicism, with some the loftiest system of morals, has in time come to stand for the acme of pride and unnaturalness.[51] So Montaigne concludes his *Apologie de Raimond Sebond* with the warning that if man wants to rise above himself *c'est à nôtre foi Chrétienne, non à sa vertu Stoique de prétendre à cette divine et miraculeuse métamorphose*, whilst Wieland,[52] equally feeling that the Stoic self-sufficiency 'departs very widely from nature' and 'can be possible only in God' adds: *Ebenso wenig konnte ich die Unterdrückung des sinnlichen Teils unseres Wesens mit der Natur reimen.* This development manifests itself in the repudiation and loss of (the obviously irrational) instincts, contempt of or hostility to woman, homosexuality,[53] and —symbol of the final victory of the *ratio* over the most basic of all instincts—the stoic glorification of suicide. With an admirable instinct Milton has seized on this phenomenon:

> Eve, *thy contempt of life and pleasure seems*
> *To argue in thee somthing more sublime*
> *And excellent then what thy mind contemnes;*
> *But self-destruction therefore saught, refutes*
> *That excellence thought in thee, and implies*
> *Not thy contempt, but anguish and regret*
> *For loss of life and pleasure overlov'd.*
>
> *P.L.* x. 1013–19

—a criticism which almost literally anticipates that of Schopenhauer.

Nevertheless Milton's ambivalence is strongly felt here. In fact, it must be doubted whether Milton ever really outgrew his earlier, Platonic self, and whether there did not remain in the recesses of his soul some misgivings and a bad conscience. Of the *Comus* period we know that he regarded chastity as 'the essential means by which the human soul reaches out to divinity',[54] whilst in *Paradise Regained* he is

49. Newton, quoting Thyer. 50. Bohn.

51. See Chap. 4 of Professor Lovejoy's *Essays in the History of Ideas* (1948).

52. *Theages*, 1760, quoted by Lovejoy, *op. cit.*, p. 68. 53. Cf. p. 34.

54. Tillyard, *op. cit.*, p. 379. For the application of this theory of Milton to his poetic creativity, see B. Rajan: 'Simple, Sensuous and Passionate', *R.E.S.* xxi (1945), 289–301, particularly pp. 299–300.

raving against Stoicism and Greek philosophy through the mouth of a hyper-stoic Jesus.[55] Inversely, the permanent bad conscience of the Greeks, their knowledge that

> *. . . who aspires must down as low*
> *as high he soard*
>
> *P.L.* ix. 169–70

and their fear of *hubris* as *the* sin, never departed from him. Thus Milton continually harps on 'inordinate pride', and deeply aware of the futility of all Icarus-flights, relegates its victims to the Paradise of Fools.[56]

More generally it has been recognized that poetic elaborations of Satan's pride and fall have always heavily drawn on classical *hubris* myths, particularly in ages when people could take it for granted that these myths, as well as those about the giants and Titans warring with Zeus, were degenerate and paganized remnants of the 'historical' Christian version, originally known to all descendants of Adam.[57] The proximity of the themes, which can easily make the one serve as allegory for the other, has been curiously demonstrated by Vondel. Vondel not only wrote a *Lucifer* and an *Adam in Exile*, but also a *Phaeton or Reckless Temerarity* (1663)[58] and a *Salmoneus* (1654).[59] More than anyone else Vondel was alive to the difference between hallowed story and pagan myth. In the *Berecht* to his *Lucifer* he writes:

'Nobody who understandeth the language of the unerring oracles of the Divine Spirit, shall judge that we indite a composition of Salmoneus, who in the mid of Elis, on his chariot and iron bridge, defying Jove and counterfeiting with a burning torch his lightning and thunder, was struck down by a bolt—neither do we rehearse an old fable of the Titan

55. Cf. pp. 88–9, 90.

56. *P.L.* iii. 466–73.

57. Cf. *P.L.* i. 740–8. Cf. also Davis P. Harding, *Milton and the Renaissance Ovid* (1946). Discussing the Satan of *P.L.*, Harding says: 'To accommodate the character and fate of Lucifer to human understanding and to make the action . . . more . . . convincing, Milton called in the aid of classical mythology' (p. 85). He discusses some of the 'pride and ambition' passages, and such names as, e.g., Typhon or Phaeton, pointing out that tradition had associated Typhon with Lucifer, and Aetna with hell (pp. 85–7). Moreover, Harding draws attention to the 'method of silent appropriation' of material from pagan myths, in addition to the ordinary allegorical use of mythology. In particular he finds Phaeton lurking behind various passages. See also D. Bush, *Mythology and the Renaissance Tradition in English Poetry* (1932), pp. 240–4, and particularly for Milton, pp. 277–8.

58. Lucifer's fall, *Isa.* xiv. 12, is also compared to Phaeton by those who, following Willamowitz, regard both as nature myths, representing the morning star superseded by the sun. Cf. Gunkel, *Schöpfung und Chaos*, pp. 132 ff.; Zimmern, *Keilinschriften und das Alte Testament*, 565 A. 7. 3; and Roscher's *Lexicon* 3. 2, col. 2201.

59. Cf. Vergil, *Aen.* vi. 585–94.

War, in the garb of which poetry endeavoured to wean its audience of reckless arrogance and ungodly sacrilege. . . .'

But nevertheless he prefixed as motto to his *Lucifer Aen.* vi. 594,[60] and when the Amsterdam magistrates capitulated to the Calvinist clergy and prohibited the *Lucifer* after two successful performances, Vondel met the emergency with a mythological master-trick. He at once composed his *Salmoneus*, the story of the King of Elis who 'aspired to deification', and produced a stage-substitute for Lucifer. Clearly the Greek king had been lurking behind the fallen archangel as his mythological shadow.[61]

Milton's profound distrust of pure spirituality links him with the Biblical world. His 'asinine Hebraism' never lets loose: he glorifies marriage and goes out of his way to denounce Stoicism in an ill-natured and querulous attack which betrays the psychological tensions and dangerous sympathies at the bottom.[62] *Samson Agonistes*, though it offers no synthesis, at least shows some approach towards one; but prior to it Milton had to follow his usual method of attempting illusory solutions by quaint intellectual gymnastics.

'By making pride (*hubris*) that which precedes disaster and self-knowledge the means of averting it, Milton is one with the Greeks. I do not think he was merely inserting Greek habits of thought because he had chosen [in *S.A.*] the Greek form of tragedy. He has a true kinship . . .' says Dr. Tillyard,[63] but goes on to quote Hanford:

'The antique strain in Milton's experience and thought stands side by side with the Christian, and the two alternate and combine in their domination of his artistic moods. It is vain that he repudiates stoicism as a futile refuge and a false philosophy, he is betrayed by the vehemence of his declarations against it, and he instinctively adopts its weapons.'

Sir Herbert Grierson, being more given to the habit of understatement, very cautiously feels, at reading the *Paradise Regained* passage referred to, that 'it is difficult not to suspect some inner conflict'.[64]

60. *praecipitemque immani turbine adegit.*

61. Vondel affords still another instance of the relation between *hubris* and the flight symbol, an example particularly moving because coming from a simple and devout Catholic who had chosen the side of obedience. In 1670, after the death of his second grandchild, he had said to his daughter: 'What is death an ugly vulture! There lyeth this fair youth and is a corpse that rotteth.' When later, after the death of his daughter Anna, he said to Agnes Block: 'Pray for me, that the Lord may take me from this life', she retorted: 'Do you want then this "ugly vulture" to come?' Vondel answered: 'Yes, let it come. For though I wait, Eliah's chariot shall not come. One has to go the common way!'

62. *P.R.* iv. 285 ff. 63. *Op. cit.*, p. 351. 64. *Op. cit.*, p. 135.

Having discussed in this chapter so many apparently irrelevant subjects as *hubris*, the Baälim, Stoicism, etc., it may seem advisable to sum up very briefly what I have tried to say and what I have not said.

In the first place I do not claim that the *hubris*-theme is *the* subject, conscious or unconscious, of *Paradise Lost*. There has been no question in this chapter of surface and esoteric meanings at all. I only contend that the *hubris*-problem is the presupposed reality, a sort of resonance-box, to the events in *Paradise Lost* and to the actions of its main protagonist. With the later poems, *hubris* emerges more distinctly, and comes to the fore as a clearly discernible centre of conflict. This is borne out by the texts, as well as by what we know of Milton's life and personality. His pride and humility, asceticism and affirmation of senses, his Old Testament and New Testament attitudes, his Graeco-Biblical ambivalence, are all clearly reflected in the ambivalence with which he treats his themes. I have chosen Stoicism as a particularly instructive example of the structure of this ambivalence and of the acuteness of the conflict caused by it.

However, one important aspect of *hubris* has been ignored so far: that overstepping one's bounds and limits implies overstepping into the bounds of another, higher being. Here *hubris* becomes *sin* in the religious sense of the word; it is gathered up into the relation of man with God, disturbing and troubling it. The Christian tradition has expressed this awareness in its accounts of the fall. The Greeks have done so in what Preller called the profoundest and most fruitful of all Greek myths: the myth of Prometheus.

Chapter Three

ANTAGONIST OF HEAVEN'S ALMIGHTY KING

MILTON's Satan has often been compared to Prometheus, and practically every critic has at least once used the epithet 'Promethean' to describe some of Satan's qualities. Already Newton had noted the affinity in his note to *Paradise Lost*, i. 94 ff.: 'Milton in this and other passages, where he is describing the fierce and unrelenting spirit of Satan, seems very plainly to have copied after the picture that Aeschylos gives of Prometheus.' He and the other commentators have pointed out various references which will in part be mentioned here. Again, Shelley[1] was greatly affected by the similarity of the two characters, clearly identifying them to a certain extent. Amongst the moderns, the best-known statement is that in Raleigh's *Milton*:[2]

'Satan unavoidably reminds us of Prometheus, and although there are essential differences, we are not made to feel them essential. His very situation as the fearless antagonist of Omnipotence makes him either a fool or a hero, and Milton is far indeed from permitting us to think him a fool. The nobility and greatness of his bearing are brought home to us in some half-dozen of the finest poetic passages in the world.'

More recently, Mr. G. R. Hamilton distinguishes between the two,[3] precisely because he feels their strong affinity. '. . . behind the tragic darkness of Satan, powerful and boasting in his own power, we catch the vision, not quite eclipsed, of an ardent Lucifer in a Heaven more truly harmonious, giving glory to Love and a world of Light.'[4]

The reactions these evaluations have called forth from modern critics have been recorded and discussed in Chapter 1. But to my knowledge the comparison has so far never been taken seriously and in a literal sense, in fact I doubt whether it was ever meant to be taken so. All that was implied by the analogy was a vague sense of the heroic at

1. Preface to *Prometheus Unbound*. See also Macaulay's essay.
2. p. 133.
3. *Op. cit.*, p. 37.
4. *Ibid.*, p. 41.

its limits: fighting not against heavy odds but against divine omnipotence itself. As a dramatic necessity, and to prevent the heroism from turning into folly,[5] the absoluteness of this omnipotence must somehow be mitigated, but this does not detract essentially from the hero's glory. Moreover, we are supposed to see in Prometheus merely a hero, the idealized struggle of mankind, and not a sinner. Says Mr. Hamilton: 'The rebellion . . . of a Prometheus, not of a Satan: a rebellion founded on the principle of love, not of self-seeking and personal ambition.'[6] The comparison thus carries a very dangerous *sous-entendu*, a critical shift of emphasis. It tends to slur over the heinous wickedness and abysmal evil of Satan, by throwing into relief his heroic virtues. Shelley, like Mr. Hamilton, was clearly aware of this, and consequently tried to delimit the two characters from each other. For that reason, too, the anti-Satanists have always rejected the comparison, which has thus become the sole property of the 'romantic' school.[7]

I doubt whether this conventional account is correct, although it is extremely revealing. It shows that we have reached a stage where the most 'unromantic' critics, while strictly adhering to the orthodox condemnation of Satan, nevertheless exhibit a markedly positive and 'romantic' response to the figure of Prometheus.[8] I almost feel certain that Hesiod himself, in contrast to Mr. Lewis or Professor Musgrove, would not have taken exception to the comparison. But he would have been deeply shocked by the words of Mr. Hamilton. Quite simply because in his eyes Prometheus would be as sinful as Satan is in the eyes of Mr. Lewis. I therefore think it worth our while to push the analogy a little further and to investigate beyond the superficial resemblance the possibility of profounder mythical, i.e., archetypal identities. I suggest that we may discover some distinctly Promethean features in the Satan of *Paradise Lost*, and that these may go a long way to explain some of the poem's major difficulties.

I do not assert, of course, that Milton consciously thought of Prometheus when describing his Satan, or that he worked Aeschylean

5. The problem of heroism and folly actually deserves a special study. It seems as if heroism, at least a certain very widespread conception of it, can never be far away from folly. That is also why the unheroic attitude is at times not cowardly but realistic. Cf., e.g., p. 9.

6. Hamilton, *op. cit.*, p. 37.

7. To which we should also reckon Schiller. See the highly interesting quotations in Mario Praz, *op. cit.*, p. 57. On the Promethean aspect see also Rex Warner's introduction to his translation of the *Prometheus Bound* (The Bodley Head, London, 1947), pp. 8–10.

8. A good example of the 'romantic' interpretation of Prometheus can be found in P. de Saint Victor's *Les Deux Masques* (3rd ed., 1883), vol. i, Chaps. 9 and 10.

references into his text in the way he did with Scripture. The actual quotations from and references to Aeschylos are relatively negligible, and certainly do not excel in quantity or significance the far more numerous allusions to Homer, Vergil, Ovid, Tasso and the like. The literal parallels[9] pointed out by the various commentators and editors such as Thyer, Richardson, Todd, Newton, Mitford and others are of small or no account here, and there is no reason to suppose any special 'influence' on Milton of Aeschylos' *Prometheus*. Fortunately so, one almost feels tempted to add, as these influences, so dear to research scholars all over the world, are usually more exact than significant. As the great Swiss scholar, the late Professor Fehr of Zürich, once put it:[10] '. . . *nachweisbare Einflüsse deuten immer nur auf das Nebensächliche, nie auf das Wesentliche hin*'. Milton owes little to Aeschylean mythology,[11] but the comparison is interesting because their myths are similar and the same archetypes seem active with both of them.

More interesting, though often too obvious to be of value, are those similarities which give us something of a common atmosphere. Such are, e.g., the identification of a God who excels mainly by his more powerful thunder

> . . . *so much the stronger prov'd*
> *He with his Thunder*
>
> P.L. i. 92–3

> . . . *he*
> *Whom Thunder hath made greater*
>
> *Ibid.*, 257–8

with Zeus:

> *The Father's thunder-clap and lightning-flame*
>
> *Prom.* 1049

> *So now let him cast, if it please him, the two-*
> *Edged curl of his lightning*
>
> *Ibid.*, 1075–6

> *The reverberant thunder is heard from the deep,*
> *And the forked flame flares of the lightning*
>
> *Ibid.*, 1116–17

9. E.g. 'adamantine chains', *P.L.* i. 48 with *Prom.* 6; 'Arimaspian', *P.L.* ii. 945 with *Prom.* 831; 'flaming sun', *P.L.* viii. 162 with *Prom.* 817. Phrases and similes like the 'proud steed reind', *P.L.* iv. 858–60 with *Prom.* 1041–2 (almost literally translated); 'spite with spite', *P.L.* ix. 178 with *Prom.* 1002; etc.

10. 'Typologische Literaturbetrachtung', *Englische Studien*, lxiv (1929).

11. Cf. C. G. Osgood, *The Classical Mythology of Milton's English Poems* (1900), pp. xlii–xliii.

(though this parallel is not confined to the Zeus of Aeschylos), and the belief in the possibility of beating God at his own game:

... when to meet the noise
Of his Almighty Engin he shall hear
Infernal Thunder, and for Lightning see
Black fire and horror shot with equal rage

P.L. ii. 64–7

Such is the wrestler he now trains against
Himself, a prodigy unconquerable,
Whose strength shall battle down the lightning blast
And master the mighty roar of heaven's thunder

Prom. 952–5

and similar points of contact.

There are however a few passages in Aeschylos which, whether sources or not, certainly evince a related pattern of emotive reaction and dramatic attitude. To these belong in the first place those passages which have been primarily responsible for the making of the comparison, those namely which express indomitable courage and unshakeable resolve. Thus Newton's note quoted above was prompted by *Paradise Lost*, i. 94 ff. as compared with

... and dost thou think that I
In fear of these new gods will cower and quake?
Far, far am I from that.

Prom. 991–3

So, let him hurl his sulphurous flames from heaven,
With white-winged snow and subterranean thunder
Make chaos and confusion of the world!
Not thus will he constrain my tongue to tell
By whose hand he from tyrrany shall fall.

Ibid., 1024–8

and by

... To bow and sue for grace
With suppliant knee, and deifie his power,
Who from the terrour of this Arm so late
Doubted his Empire, that were low indeed,
That were an ignominy and shame beneath
This downfall

P.L. i. 111–16

as compared with

Or dost thou deem that I, fearing the purpose
Of Zeus, will, woman-hearted, supplicate
My hated adversary with bow abased
And abject inclination of my palms,
To free me from my bondage?

Prom. 1034–8

The satanic solution of the problem of liberty and service, discussed on p. 37, has its counterpart in *Prom.* 998–9

I have no wish to change my adverse fortune,
Be well assured, for thy subservience

and Newton was probably right in suggesting that Milton intended to answer this with Abdiel's Christian

Reign thou in Hell thy Kingdom, let mee serve
In Heav'n God ever blest, and his Divine
Behests obey, worthiest to be obey'd.

P.L. vi. 183–5

What greatly strengthens the resemblance is the divine, or rather semi-divine nature of the protagonists in both cases. The contest is inflated to enormous dimensions by the fact that none of the parties can, properly speaking, be annihilated. The knowledge of at least the possibility of immortality is a decisive factor of Satan's resistance:

. . . *since by Fate the strength of Gods*
And this Empyreal substance cannot fail

Ibid., i. 116–17

. . . *laid thus low,*
As far as Gods and Heav'nly Essences
Can perish

Ibid., 137–9

Since now we find this our Empyreal form
Incapable of mortal injurie
Imperishable

Ibid., vi. 433–5

even as with Prometheus

What should I fear, predestined not to die

Prom. 965

For with death I cannot be stricken.

Ibid., 1086

With this impossibility of dying should be compared *P.L.* ii. 95 ff. and the idea of death as a desirable impossibility *P.L.* x. 775 ff. and 783 ff., together with the fragment of the *Prometheus Lyomenos* preserved by Cicero[12]

amore mortis terminum anquirens mali.

Here the sufferings of Prometheus have reached such a pitch of intensity, that immortality, instead of being a source of hope, has become hell

. . . where peace
And rest can never dwell, hope never comes
That comes to all

P.L. i. 65–7

to him that had brought hope to all:

First I implanted in his heart blind hopes,

Prom. 266

Equally underlying both actions is the assumed possibility of overthrowing Jove's order. For Satan

. . . endanger'd Heav'ns perpetual King;
And put to proof his high supremacy

P.L. i. 131–2

God himself being gravely concerned about his omnipotence.

Let us advise, and to this hazard draw
With speed what force is left, and all imploy
In our defence, lest unawares we lose
This our high place.

P.L. v. 729–32

Prometheus, suffering his time

Decreed till Zeus from tyranny hath fallen

Prom. 782

is sustained by the knowledge that even

He [*Zeus*] *could not alter that which is ordained*

Ibid., 534

And yet shall Zeus, so obstinate of spirit,
Be humbled. . . .

Ibid., 939 ff.

12. *Tusc. Disp.* ii. 10.

These are, I believe, all the external resemblances between the *Prometheus Desmotes* and *Paradise Lost*. Individually they are not astounding, nor is their cumulative evidence in any way telling. Even the points of resemblance mentioned last, although they go deeper, do not reveal their significance at a mere visual inspection. It is necessary first to state who Prometheus is and what the Promethean myth may mean, before one can hope to extract the full value of the comparison. Only with a right understanding of this myth is it possible to read the texts with their full resonance. I do not suggest that by then we shall have discovered an identity of the Lucifer and Prometheus myths, or that the Satan of *Paradise Lost* is simply a blend of the two. I merely claim at present that the Promethean myth shows a harmonious development which overlaps to a great extent that of the Christian Satan, and that by looking closer into the meaning of the former, we shall understand many things about Milton and his *Paradise Lost*.

As has already been remarked, the Promethean myth can also be read romantically, that is with an antinomian attitude. But the Prometheus of Goethe,[13] Shelley and Spitteler is not the classical one. Although the romantic readings may thus have to be discarded when we want to analyse the Greek Prometheus in a scientifically responsible manner, yet, even so, they can claim legitimate consideration. The fact alone that the original myth showed itself capable of so vital and strong a development[14] is at least as interesting as the exegesis of the Greek texts. In trying first to give a short outline of the Promethean myth, I shall therefore limit myself to a statement of the essential facts and data, in so far as they seem to me of direct relevance to our present inquiry, without going into technical detail such as, e.g., a comparison of the Hesiodic and Aeschylean versions.[15] In the first place it should be noted that the Promethean world lacks the sense of creation. Man's creatureliness, as we have it in biblical tradition, is unknown. Men and gods are coeternal and of common origin; both are children of

13. *Vermischte Gedichte. Prometheus.*

14. For the evolution of the Prometheus figure in literature, see Karl Heinemann, *Die tragischen Gestalten der Griechen in der Weltliteratur* (1920), vol. i, Chap. 2, which, though mainly concentrating on European drama (Calderon, Goethe, Shelley, Edgar Quinet, etc.), also discusses Byron, Spitteler a.o.; and Margarete Ostrowski-Sachs, 'Die Wandlungen des Prometheus-Mythus' in *Der Psychologe*, ii. 7–8 (Sonderheft zum 75. Geburtstag von C. G. Jung, 1950), pp. 334–43, a rather short but readable survey of the trend of development of the myth.

15. On Prometheus, see Roscher's *Lexicon*, 3.2, 3032–3110, and, for a recent and very profound study, Karl Kerényi, *Prometheus* (Zürich, 1946), which is a further elaboration of the interpretation given by the same author in his *Die Antike Religion*, pp. 157–62.

Gaia, in spite of all their fundamental differences.[16] They are two poles of existence. *Prima facie* man is therefore neither creature nor rebel.[17]

Secondly, Prometheus himself is a god, like Zeus. The fact that somehow he comes to stand for mankind as their suffering champion, and possibly as their type and symbol, must not make us oblivious to his essentially divine nature. As Kerényi says, Prometheus is first and foremost a god. The paradox here lies in the fact that he undergoes insult and suffering in a typically human manner. This distinguishes him both from Christ and from the romantic Prometheus. Jesus is primarily a man. In his case the paradox comes through the faith that the man Jesus is also God. The romantic Prometheus, Goethe's for instance, is man claiming the rank and dignity of God. His suffering is that of mankind, but his protest is that of outraged divinity, or rather of the divine quality of his humanity. The only parallel to Prometheus would therefore be a gnostic *Urmensch*, *anthropos* or *Adam Kadmon*.[18] In the mythological sphere Prometheus is thus the divine representative of the non-olympic, the human pole of the world.

Thirdly, the fact should be noted that Prometheus suffers during daytime. With sunrise the eagle of Zeus, itself an obvious symbol for the sun (which is actually apostrophized once by Prometheus as 'bird of Zeus'), comes to feed on his liver. Now the liver of Prometheus grows again during night. But also generally speaking the liver belongs to the night as the traditional seat of the passions, partly also because of its dark colour, and last but not least in its function as a means of divination.[19] The unbinding of Prometheus and his liberation from daylight suffering therefore correspond to an important step forward in the evolution of the human image in man. He has now become a daylight being, and is accepted as such by the gods.

This brings us back again to the problem of the development of consciousness, already discussed in the preceding chapter. The view put forward there was that the *hubris* problem was essentially one of the evolution of the human *psyche* to consciousness. The connection with the Promethean myth, based on the same problem, though dealing with it in a more inclusive and existential way, is obvious.

Already Prometheus' first and original act, as told by Hesiod[20] is one of differentiation. His second act, that to which he chiefly owes his

16. 'Of one race, one only, are men and gods; both of one mother's womb we draw our breath: but far asunder is all our power divided and parts us—here there is nought and there is strength of bronze, a seat unshaken, eternal, abides the heaven above'. (Pindar, *Nemea*, vi. 1–5). The same is said by Hesiod, *Works and Days*, 108. See also Kerényi, *op. cit.*, pp. 13–15.

17. See Chapter 5, note 3.

18. Kerényi, *op. cit.*, pp. 9 and 54–5.

19. *Ibid.*, pp. 22–3.

20. *Theogony*, 535 ff.

fame, the bringing of fire, equally points to a *prise de conscience* symbolism. It is unnecessary, indeed it would be impossible here, to mention all the evidence and literature on the subject. The best-known example probably is the descent of the Holy Ghost, visible as 'cloven tongues like as of fire'. But also in Greek philosophy, from Heraclitus to the Stoics, fire and its qualities were a favourite subject of speculation. Empedocles ascribed to fire consciousness, thought and knowledge, qualities which Heraclitus thought were a divine prerogative, whilst Aristotle allowed them to men also, though admitting their divine provenance.[21] For if there is anything divine in man, it is undoubtedly his consciousness of himself, whether we call it soul, spirit, reason or thought. Its most prominent symptom is the loss of man's original unity, or even identity with the world. The primitive *participation mystique* has given way to a new distance of man not only towards nature, but also towards himself. Man has ceased to exist as a mere piece of nature, something has emerged within him in virtue of which he now stands over and above himself and the world. Life in its specifically human sense, as thought, speech, purposeful and creative activity, is the expression of man's new status and dignity. But every light has its shadow—even as every shadow has its light—and to every medal there is a reverse. *Homo sapiens* is not only given mastery over the world as *homo faber*[22] and exercising dominion over 'the fish of the sea, and over the fowl of the air, and over every living thing that moveth upon earth'. He is also harassed by a new uneasiness and a new sense of guilt and danger. Original unity and *participation mystique* may be characteristic of a low level of psychic evolution, but at any rate they imply living in a stable and integrated community with a greater and more embracing, albeit less conscious whole. The way of individuation, however, and the growth towards consciousness and freedom is a process of severance from this original unity, and is attended accordingly by feelings of uneasiness and loneliness.[23] The image that obtrudes itself is, of course, that of human birth and of the embryonic organism exchanging the security of the motherly body for a more individual existence, exposed to greater dangers. This image is more than a comparison. It is, as experience has shown, a real archetype. To speak here figuratively of a birth-trauma may therefore be misleading. Perhaps it would be better to regard the birth-trauma as the most concrete and obvious example and therefore also the most ready-at-

21. See Ostrowski-Sachs, *art. cit.*, p. 335.
22. On intelligence and the *homo faber* see Henri Bergson, *L'Evolution Créatrice* 62nd ed., (1946), pp. 138 ff.
23. Cf. p. 30.

hand symbol of this aspect of the pattern of life. Every dimension stretches into two directions, and every 'birth' opens a new dimension of life. It is only appropriate that man's new sensibilities should also give him the possibility of negative experiences,[24] and that anxiety, care, unhappiness, injustice and spiritual suffering should rear their ugly heads in the newly opened vistas.

Another danger of increasing consciousness is that it may lead to a feeling of equality with the gods through the awareness that one shares their knowledge, freedom and power. Together with consciousness there emerges thus a sense of guilt and sin. The double consequence is that on the one hand man himself does not want to be free,[25] and on the other, that the gods too look askance at every human attempt to reach out towards higher levels of personality. A third corollary is the rather queer position of religion in this scheme: it is a system of behaviour where man respects and serves his jealous gods, carefully avoiding offence by anything that might look like independence, freedom, or self-consciousness. Literary illustrations are legion; but one thinks in the first place of Nietzsche, though one may also cite Spitteler's *Prometheus*, Quinet's trilogy[26] *Prometheus*, Dostoievski's Great Inquisitor, and, for a modern variation on the same theme, Jean-Paul Sartre's play *Les Mouches*. The hybridic shadow of every new progress of knowledge makes it a boon and a bane at the same time, a victory and a punishment, a double-edged sword—like that mysterious element, fire. It is a blessing, but can also be destruction if it is not carefully limited and kept down. But significantly enough it is also the only element whose natural tendency is upwards. Moreover, like the spirit, it confers might and mastery, and with the fire at his disposal, nature becomes mere raw-material in the hands of man, who in his turn becomes shaper and creator. Fire is the appropriate symbol for the spirit and knowledge which is in man and by which he 'aspires to divinity' and becomes a god.[27] It is therefore quite in order that the bringer of

24. For the relation of this profound psychological ambivalence to cultural and sociological problems, and in particular to our modern crisis, see E. Fromm, *The Fear of Freedom*, (1945).

25. Cf. Fromm, *op. cit.*

26. 1883. A short account of the two last mentioned can be found in Heinemann, *op. cit.*, pp. 37 and 32.

27. The other alternative for man would be to conceive of himself *a priori* as created in God's image. In the Biblical sphere man's protection against the danger of hybridic inflation and arrogated god-like mastery over nature, would be the institution of the Sabbath. That the commandment not only of rest, but negatively of abstention from work (*Exod.* xx. 10; *Deut.* v. 14; *Exod.* xxxi. 13–15, xxxv. 2) is a literally 'religious' self-limitation before the Lord of All, is clearly brought out by the juxtaposed motivations: because God is the creator of the world (*Exod.* xx. 11,

fire is called—*nomen est omen*—Prometheus, the 'knower', or, to be more precise, the 'foreknower', although in his relations with Zeus he proved himself an Epimetheus:

Falsely we named thee the Foresighted One,
Prometheus—thine the need of foresight now,
How from this art to extricate thyself!

Prom. 85–7

It is of course possible that the two brothers were originally one undifferentiated being. But more important for our present purpose than his probably different and less transparent original name or names, is the fact that he ended as a *Prometheus*. It is his knowledge which determines his actions, which made him side with Zeus in the Titan war and which gave him security in his perseverance against Zeus.

But Prometheus has more than knowledge. He has cunning. He is astute and clever, and Zeus himself had profited from his 'smartness' not less than mankind.[28] But this astuteness implies, as Kerényi points out,[29] a certain crookedness of mind, ranging from deceitfulness to inventiveness. Prometheus is *ankulometes*, that is, his thinking is *ankulos*, crooked—the mark of a basic deficiency which wants to be overcome. Zeus, the god, whose being knows no inherent defections, *per definitionem* lacks this crookedness, and may thus well need at times the help of a Prometheus.

The order of Zeus is perfect, regulated and static. His world has measure and limits, and every being is assigned its place. But, and here the trouble starts, the human pole of the universe, as soon as it becomes aware of itself at all, becomes aware of fatal deficiencies. Man's attempt to cope with this situation by remedying these deficiencies, presupposes a mental make-up foreign to Zeus. Cleverness is a compensatory function of defectiveness, and man's resourcefulness is thus the means

xxxi. 17) and because Israel was a servant in the land of Egypt whence they were brought out through a mighty hand and a stretched-out arm (*Deut.* v. 15), the corollary obviously being that 'unto me the children of Israel are servants; they are my servants whom I have brought forth out of the land of Egypt: I am the Lord your God'. (*Lev.* xxv. 55). For the rest all the learned critical disquisitions on the double motivation of the Sabbath-law are completely besides the point. As further evidence of the relation of the Sabbath to the Promethean problem, one might add that the prohibition of work is always couched in general terms without any detail: 'Thou shalt not do any work', with but one notable exception: 'Ye shall kindle no fire throughout your habitations upon the sabbath day' (*Exod.* xxxv. 3). Cf. also pp. 63–4.

28. Hesiod, *Theogony*, 540, 546, 701, etc., Aesch. *Prom.*, 215 ff.

29. *Op. cit.*, pp. 20–21 and 56.

by which he evades and oversteps the rules and bounds set by Zeus, whilst Zeus, like Milton's God, may ironically look on. Kerényi's comment on *Theogony*, 550–2:[30] '*Durchschauend den Trug lässt er* [Zeus] *sich belisten, doch nicht überlisten.... Er enthält das Sein impliziert und unbeweglich, die Taten und Untaten mit ihren Folgen, kennt daher auch gar kein Wünschen und Aendernwollen*' might be equally said of Milton's God, and almost sounds like a paraphrase of *P.L.* iii. 77 ff., but particularly of God's words:

> *... be not dismaid,*
> *Nor troubl'd at these tidings from the Earth,*
> *Which your sincerest care could not prevent,*
> *Foretold so lately what would come to pass,*
> *When first this Tempter cross'd the Gulf from Hell.*
> *I told ye then he should prevail and speed*
> *On his bad Errand....*
>
> *P.L.* x. 35–41

Prometheus thus betrays some essentially human characteristics. In fact, he is the founder of human existence as specifically human: he invented the sacrifice and brought the fire. The latter raised the fireless animal existence to the level of the human. Everything now changes into the specifically human, even man's vulnerability. He no longer suffers dumbly, anonymously, as a part of nature, but existentially, as a human. He questions himself and the universe, he calls the world to witness, he measures reality against another ideal order, in short, he can suffer unjustly. His suffering is doubled by becoming the direct source of a further suffering, that of the spirit: man suffers from the injustice of his suffering, because, from *his* standpoint, his actions were necessary and unavoidable. In the case of Prometheus, his actions were prompted by his adopting the human point of view, by his love and friendship for mankind:

> *Yet of my present state I cannot speak*
> *Cannot be silent. The gifts I gave to man*
> *Have harnessed me beneath this harsh duress.*
>
> . . . . .
>
> *Such the transgressions which I expiate,*
> *A helpless captive....*
>
> *Prom.* 106 ff.

Herein lies the daring of the Greek tragedian, which in many respects even outdoes that of the author of the book of Job.

30. *Op. cit.*, p. 30.

O majestical mother, O heavenly Sky,
In whose region revolveth the Light of the World,
Thou seest the Wrongs that I suffer![31]

Prom. 1125–7

are the words with which Prometheus disappears in Tartaros.

It is this aspect of the Promethean drama which so strongly appeals to us that we forget that Prometheus is actually trespassing, violating Zeus' order, the *dike*. For if we recognize in Prometheus our own existential suffering, we must equally recognize that this is due primarily to his specifically human sin. *Sin* as the violation of Zeus' order in an attempt to supplement a deficiency, and specifically *human* in the sense that both the awareness of this deficiency and the idea and resolve to overcome it, are peculiar to human existence, that is consciousness. Prometheus has been guilty of *hubris* by ignoring his limits in a very profound sense. He is accused that

A god, thou didst defy the wrath of gods,
On men their powers bestowing beyond due. [Literally: beyond their *dike*]

Prom. 29–30

and himself admits as much in similar, though at the same time vitally different words:

For my too great *love of the children of men.*

Prom. 124

But this 'beyond measure' is, humanly speaking, a bare minimum. For what the original *dike* of Zeus would have meant to men, has been made clear by Hesiod[32] and Aeschylos:

No sooner was he on his father's throne
. . . but held the hapless race of man
Of no account, resolving to destroy
All human kind and sow new seed on earth.
And none defied his will in this save me,
I dared to do it, I delivered man
From death and steep destruction.

Prom. 244 ff.

The *basso continuo* of the Promethean drama is thus given: the inevitability of trespassing. Trespassing, because no one thinks of denying Zeus' exclusive right to dispose of the fire at his own discretion;

31. Or: 'Thou seest how unjustly I suffer.'
32. *Works and Days*, 42–6.

inevitable, because without Prometheus' theft the human race would have perished.[33]

We are now far enough to summarize the main implications of the Promethean myth as presented by Aeschylos or as interpreted later, often in variance to, but always in organic development from, the Aeschylean meaning. These are:

In the first place a sense of deficiency, even of fatal deficiency, inherent in human existence, and consequently a constitutive factor of the human *prise de conscience*.

Secondly, man's attempt to remedy this state of affairs is a manifestation of dynamism which violates the static harmony, order and *dike* of the cosmic household, whose norm and law is the will of Father Zeus.

Thirdly, human suffering is conceived as the inevitable concomitant of the equally inevitable wrongdoing. It gains moreover a specifically human depth of agony by being doubled in the sufferer's consciousness by becoming a suffering of injustice, if not yet a suffering for the sake of righteousness. Existence is seen as the tragic equation of 'action is suffering', though not yet of 'suffering is action'.

Fourthly, the idea of transcendence, by which I mean the extra-human reality, the 'other' pole: heaven and the gods, is necessarily conceived as personified world-order, impersonal fate, a cold and hard omnipotence.[34] It is essential to keep this in mind. For in spite of his anthropomorphic behaviour, his irascibility and revengefulness, Zeus is here rather impersonal, cold and aloof. For our appreciation of the character of Zeus in his relations with Prometheus, i.e., mankind, it is immaterial to define his precise relation to Fate and

The three-formed Moires and the remembering Erinies.

Prom. 532

Actually this relation changes and develops in the drama, and one of the main interests of Aeschylos is the evolution of Zeus and of his manner of government, and the final consolidation of his order.[35] But all this is outside the scope of our present purpose. What matters here is the fact that the Zeus whom Prometheus opposes is dangerously near the Father of *Paradise Lost*, or rather that the God of *Paradise Lost*

33. This was clearly the intention of Zeus. It should be noted, however, that according to one possible interpretation, Prometheus' solicitude for mankind, which overlooked its essential limitations, frustrated the purpose of Zeus which was (Hesiod) to create another, more permanent race after this one had passed away. (*Aesch. Prom.*, 247–9.) Because of Prometheus, humanity survives in permanent and irreparable limitations. The myth might consequently be described as a sort of theodicy.

34. *Prom.*, 156–9, 173–4.

35. Cf. note 7 to Chapter 6.

is dangerously near the Zeus of the Greek drama.[36] The difference between the two lies not with God, but with his opponents: Prometheus suffers in his own sphere

See what I suffer from the gods, a god!

Prom. 92

whilst Satan sets himself up as a sort of anti-god.

These observations bring us back to the considerations of the preceding chapter. Even as the Greek *hubris* is a dynamic movement of man, by definition conceived as inordinate and as an encroachment, so the action of Prometheus too is an encroachment on the limits imposed on man. Bertrand Russell's definition of *hubris* should be recalled here: 'Where there is vigour, there is a tendency to overstep just bounds.' The punishment that follows *hubris* (*nemesis*) 'restores the eternal order which the aggressor sought to violate'.[37] *Human* consciousness, and its consequence, *human* action, are as such inordinate, a 'too much', a sinful aspiration and rebellious trespass. We are at the point where civilization and culture, which are human consciousness, resourcefulness and power in action, inevitably take on the character of hybridic trespass. The archetypal structure is given which, in certain circumstances and under the influence of certain ideas, can lead to the rather quietistic attitude which we shall find to be inherent in Christianity.

There is of course still another way, which is, however, apt to become a full-fledged antinomianism. It is the way of making a virtue of necessity, and has been chosen by the so-called romantics. Prometheus is now recognized as the prototype of humanity and its few heroes. On this premise it matters little whether the Promethean action and suffering are bewailed as a tragic necessity or exultingly glorified as the apotheosis of heroism. In any case the borderline into the Satanic has been crossed. This can be done with the naïve and ardent idealism of a Shelley, which tries to put itself at ease by distinguishing between Satan's heinous wickedness and Prometheus' virtuous self-sacrifice for humanity; as well as with Blake's thoroughly perverse glorification of passionate energy and his hybridic repudiation of all bounds and limits. Equally characteristic is Saint-Victor's rapturous rhapsody on the history of civilization as a perpetuation of the Promethean crime.[38] For him, as for all romantics, Prometheus incarnates the genius of mankind. He lives in all the great moments of human progress. He is Roger

36. See also Grierson, *op. cit.*, pp. 105 ff. It should be noted in this connection that the 'divine irony' so much talked about by Milton-critics is actually the same thing as the 'homeric' laughter of the Greek gods. On the latter see Kerényi, *Die Antike Religion*, pp. 163 ff.

37. *Op. cit.*, pp. 134–5.

38. *Op. cit.*, pp. 339–42.

Bacon, Averroës, Galileo and Giordano Bruno, always victim of the jealousy of the gods and the ingratitude of men. *Le Titan est puni de ses bienfaits, châtié de ses dons; il expia sa science par la souffrance et son génie par la dérision.*[39] Man's agony, victory and despair in his struggle against the iron laws of a superior fate, indifferently dispensing good and evil, is symbolized by Prometheus who is *le prophète permanent, la voix inextinguible de ses cris de l'âme.*[40] The stage of his efforts may have outwardly changed, but *ses bourreaux le torturent sous d'autres masques et par d'autres fers; d'autres aigles se relaient sur sa plaie incessamment élargie. Mais Eschyle reconnaitrait encore son Titan dans ce Prométhée transformé qui n'est autre que l'homme éternel.*[41]

I have quoted at some length not only because these passages seem fairly representative of the romantic mind, but mainly because of the conclusions they lead up to. It is the refusal, already to be found in Shelley, to agree to the traditional solution of the drama, and to accept the 'sham peace' imposed on Aeschylos by Greek religious tradition. No, Prometheus perseveres in his revolt and suffering. *Le temps, en détruisant le Prométhée Délivré, a revoqué sa grâce souscrite par Eschyle. Il ne connaît que le Prométhée Enchaîné, il n'admire et il ne comprend que lui seul* . . .[42] Curiously enough, this attitude (Goethe's, Shelley's) recoils from an all-round identification with Satan. Whether this is due to an intuition of the evitability of this identification, or to mere fear, I would not decide here. Suffice it to note that there were others who did not recoil: Blake, Byron and Nietzsche, and that the accusation of devil-worship addressed to the romantics is not quite without foundation.[43]

But the case of Shelley and his similars shows that there is another side to the picture. Mention has already been made of differences between Prometheus and Christ. But these also imply the existence of resemblances: the god who throws in his lot with mankind, who takes upon himself the existential suffering of a humanity otherwise doomed to perdition, or at least to a hopeless impasse, and therefore in vital need of succour, liberation and salvation. *Prometheus* ll. 702–74 are unique in classical Greek literature. They are the expectation of a saviour! The analogy becomes still more significant when we consider the role of vicarious suffering in the unbinding of Prometheus. Heracles, sheer male strength, liberates the 'foreknower' Prometheus; but also wounds with his arrow, aimed at the centaur Elatos, Cheiron, another centaur, the good and wise physician. The saviour who disappears in the underworld, taking upon himself the Promethean suffering, is the half-divine, half-animal physician, the healer who bears pain in all

39. *Op. cit.*, p. 340. 40. *Ibid.*, p. 342. 41. *Ibid.*, p. 342.
42. *Ibid.*, p. 345. 43. Cf. p. 81. See also p. 4, note 11.

eternity. No wonder, then, that in spite of the many profound differences between the two myths, the early Fathers could point to Prometheus as the symbol of Christ.[44] Tertullian[45] speaks of the *crucibus Caucasorum* and exclaims: *Verus Prometheus, deus omnipotens, blasphemiis lancinatus*, whilst others found god-and-man in a bold anagram (*Protheus*), or dilated on the similarities of the sufferings of Prometheus and the passion of Christ, comparing Zeus' eagle to the lance, the Oceanides to the disciples, Cheiron's descent to Hades with that of Christ to hell, the virgin conception of Io and of Mary, and more fond similarities of this sort.[46]

The Promethean myth thus betrays an interesting ambivalence, and shows itself capable of developing in two directions. As a typical Lucifer, 'bringer of light', Prometheus shares the full ambivalence of this archetypal image. He has a light and a dark side, which can either differentiate into two sharply distinguished figures (as has happened with the original Lucifer)[47] or else remain a multivalent, amorphous whole, lending itself, at the bid of occasion, to absorption by and amalgamation with other, more clear-cut and determined images. The Promethean myth can thus point towards Christ as well as towards Satan, according to our susceptibilities and our views about man, as imposed on us by our civilization and the exigencies of our psychic situation.

As will be shown in the next chapter, early Biblical thought is relatively unconcerned with these problems. Human activity as such is essentially god-willed, nay, even commanded, as long as the right attitude and the right proportions are guarded. To illustrate this one would have to give a phenomenological analysis of the various Biblical stories, laws, ordinances and rites connected with human activity. But even the Jewish *homo faber* lacks all Promethean emotion.[48] As the Rabbis said in the Talmud,[49] God himself created the first pair of tongs just before Sabbath eve, i.e., at the end of his six days' work, and gave them to man, because 'to make tools a first tool is needed'. This is the same God who clothed Adam and Eve[50] and instructed them further,[51] Adam qualifying in the end Cain's posterity as

44. Cf. also Shelley, *Prometheus Unbound*, Act i, ll. 578–85, and Heinemann's account of Quinet's trilogy (*op. cit.*, pp. 32–3) and of Siegfried Lipiner's epic, *Der Entfesselte Prometheus* (1875) (*ibid.*, pp. 34–5).

45. *Adv. Marc.* 1.1.

46. Saint Victor, *op. cit.*, pp. 335–7.

47. Cf. pp. 98–9.

48. On the Greek *homo faber* cf. Russell's opinion quoted on p. 29.

49. *Aboth*, v. 9.

50. *Gen.* iii. 21.

51. Cf. also *P.L.* x. 1056–62 ff.

. . . Inventers rare,
Unmindful of thir Maker, though his Spirit
Taught them, but they his gifts acknowledg'd none.

P.L. xi. 610–12

It seems not too much to say that in the question of human progress and self-assertion the pagan, i.e., Greek in Milton got the upper hand over the Hebrew. One feels that in Milton's scheme Prometheus is nearer to Satan than to Christ. After all, he is a bringer of light and as such a *lucifer*, like Satan.[52] The circumstances in which Christianity was born made it inevitable that every *lucifer* should be vehemently rejected (except, of course *ille . . . Lucifer qui nescit occasum*[53]), and that the bringing of light and fire, in fact every human surge forwards, should be abandoned for that other 'light of the world' whose passion, death, and resurrection were to supplement the dramatic 'action is suffering' with the messianic, or rather Christian, 'suffering is action'.[54] Moreover, the fact that the Son has to mediate between God the Father and mankind, tends to give the former the inhuman remoteness of Zeus, turns him into Raleigh's 'whimsical tyrant', and is also responsible for Blake's equation that with Milton 'the Father is Destiny'. M. Saurat, who heartily agrees with this,[55] quotes in support:

As they would confine th' interminable,
And tie him to his own prescript,
Who made our Laws to bind us, not himself

S.A. 307–9

lines remarkably similar to Aeschylos'

None is free but Zeus.

Prom. 50

Although the Biblical Satan, even the post-Biblical and patristic Lucifer, is the product of a very different psychic constellation than the one that produced Prometheus, there are enough inherent similarities to make contaminations and amalgamations possible. The initial develop-

52. The identification of Lucifer *Isa.* xiv. 12 with Satan, though a notorious historical error, is nevertheless a genuine and profound psychological intuition. Schärf, *op. cit.*, p. 274, note 91.

53. See p. 98–9.

54. It is the redemptive, i.e., active character of suffering which constitutes the great contribution of the Servant chapters of *Isaiah*, and which gives them that messianic quality on which later christology could legitimately draw, in spite of the orthodox exegetical nonsense which it entailed. It is this same quality which is just outside the reach of the Greek dramatist.

55. *Op. cit.*, pp. 105 and 130 ff.

ment depends on the sort of 'fatherhood' ascribed to God. It can be that of Zeus, the Olympian *pater familias*, guardian of custom, law and the present order; in other words the father-image functioning as the mediator of the (conservative) collective conscience. But it can also be that of the Biblical God, which is the transpersonal imperative for a creative change and movement towards new levels. This is the God of Abraham who said: 'Get thee out of thy country, and from thy kindred, and from thy father's house, unto the land that I will show thee'.[56] Appropriately enough, rabbinical legend tells that as a true revolutionary, Abraham, before leaving, destroyed all his father Terah's idols.[57] Historical Christianity, one must conclude, has chosen the former. The Christian acceptance of the ambivalent Greek *hubris*-complex, combined with a Hebrew sense of a calling by and relation to a personal God, could easily create a situation where every human act must be a sinful trespass,[58] and where in fact there can be no escape except the intervention of divine grace. Not only is this very different from the old Jewish idea of God, to whom the people have direct and immediate contact and who, in spite of occasional outbursts, nevertheless loves his people and yearns for them. It is tantamount to saying that every human act, as long as it is merely *human*, is hybridic, Promethean, and of the devil. In other words, every human move is condemned. The only thing that matters is Christ's move towards us, and (possibly) our response. Implicitly this contains a condemnation of civilization of which the Greek myth in itself can hardly be said to be guilty in this form, but into which its archetypal meaning could develop and be intensified, when absorbed into the Christian climate. Professor Grierson is certainly right when saying[59] that the 'pessimism' ascribed by Dr. Tillyard to Milton personally, is actually inherent in the Evangelicism of Milton's time and 'indeed . . . in Christianity in any form that is historical'.

We have by now come to understand how the hybridic Lucifer can

56. *Gen.* xii. 1.

57. Of course even the Jewish God, once having given laws and commandments, could not help becoming a conservative *pater familias* himself. Like Abraham, Jesus had to be an iconoclast and revolutionary. In due course the time came for *his* so-called successors to be the pillars of reactionary conservatism. Nevertheless, the emergence of the revolutionary, prophetic, 'calling' God, out of the Jewish unconscious, and the relatively high number of Jews in revolutionary movements of all sorts, not only partly substantiates some of the stock antisemitic contentions, but also throws a new light on their springs and basic motives.

58. Cf. the reference to Masson, p. 75. There is, I suspect, more truth in Masson's rather simplistic pseudo-psychological analysis of Lucifer, than is apparent at first sight.

59. *Op. cit.*, p. 97.

be charged with Promethean qualities. We must therefore turn again to Milton, and study to what extent he adhered to this extreme 'Barthianism', and whether the Hebrew, the Prometheus, or the 'romantic' in him did not at the same time voice his protest.

But before doing so, it will be necessary for us to outline first the Christian scheme of Milton and the place therein of the facts and problems which we have studied hitherto in their Greek garb. However vital and real these Greek myths and concepts may be for an understanding of Milton, they are, at their best, but part of the foundations or single bricks of the imposing and many-mansioned house which is Milton's Christianity. To understand Milton's poems aright it is indispensable first to isolate the centres of gravity of his Christian scheme, to explore their relation to his other ideals and aspirations (either avowed or repressed), and to determine the tensions to which they gave rise and the solutions, or lack of solutions, they led to. This quest of 'centres of gravity' may well call forth a second time the reproach of irresponsible arbitrariness, but here too I hope that the end will succeed in justifying the means.

Chapter Four

THE KINGDOM, THE POWER, AND THE GLORY

THERE are central points upon which a poem may pivot, even if its avowed purpose or surface meaning is not directly connected with them. But works of art possess an independence of their own. The texture of the verse, the meaning it conveys by its intensity, its overtones and undertones, soon develop centres of gravity of their own. To ignore these is to falsify the significance of a poem.

This does not mean that we must look for 'unconscious meanings'. I think this term one of the unhappiest coinages, not because it exaggerates the function of the poetic realities it expresses, but rather because it gives a wrong idea of their nature. In virtue of certain qualities it possesses, a poem may carry unexpected significances, but these lie in the poem itself, though ultimately grounded in the poet; whereas meanings, in any 'meaning'-ful sense of the word, can only be ascribed to the poet. *Paradise Lost* still keeps the stage, although it is a comparative failure,[1] because it contains and communicates such significances. If a work of art is to survive, it must hide 'some great human truth, some appeal to universal human aspirations, decked in the garb of symbolism. The poet himself may not be fully conscious of his deeper meaning, and the manner of its involution is something quite different from the methods of the so-called school of symbolists, but there it must be, hidden or manifest'.[2]

This principle laid down by Mr. More seems true enough; unfortunately his application of it to *Paradise Lost* is not very successful. The principle as such is, of course, the fundamental assumption of the profounder psychological approach to literature, by which I mean the approach based on the insights of C. G. Jung. Applying Jung's psychology to poetry means to look for the sources of the vitality of the works we call 'great art', to find out why they strike responsive chords

1. Cf. pp. 27–8. 2. Paul Elmer More, *Shelburne Essays*, Fourth Series, p. 240.

in us, so invariably and so powerfully; in other words, to analyse the primordial images and archetypal patterns which they contain and reawaken in the reader. The only work known to me which undertakes to investigate literary problems on these lines, is Miss Maud Bodkin's *Archetypal Patterns in Poetry* (1934).[3] In one respect it shares the fault of Mr. More's essay: the application in detail is deficient. As is to be expected in a pioneer study, occasional over-simplification, one-sided stressing of particular points together with lack of consideration for the 'literary' aspects and context of the passages analysed, and finally, a certain half-confused vagueness, at times leave the reader with a feeling of dissatisfaction, which may be due, I think, to Miss Bodkin's failure to push her analyses far enough and to delve fully into the depths of Jung's symbolism on the one hand, and on the other hand, to keep in mind systematically the more literary aspects.

The ideas of the Kingdom and the Power seem to me to be the centres of gravity of *Paradise Lost*. They correspond, in a way, to what Dr. Tillyard has called the theme of 'heroic energy'.[4] Power and might are almost obsessions with Milton;[5] his sensitivity to strength and energy burgeons out continually. Even his awareness of 'values' moral, aesthetic or religious, is determined by their power-aspect. It is not the beauty of holiness, nor the holiness of beauty that appeals to Milton; it is the power of holiness, the power of beauty, the power of goodness, that carry him away. 'Milton's stock in trade is composed not of ideas, but of energies', says Professor Wilson Knight, '. . . [he] . . . is our supreme exponent of power in all its grades'.[6] Thus when Zephon surprises Satan 'squat like a toad' at Eve's ear, his grave rebuke

> *Severe in youthful beautie, added grace*
> Invincible: *abasht the Devil stood,*
> *And felt* how awful goodness is.
>
> *P.L.* iv. 845–7[7]

3. For her discussion of Milton's Satan, one of the unsatisfactory parts of her book, cf. *ibid.*, pp. 230–45. Unfortunately I have not had access to S. E. Hyman's *The Armed Vision* (1948), where several other similar studies are discussed.

4. *Op. cit.*, pp. 279, 284, 290.

5. The significance of the power-problem with Milton has also been clearly seen by Mutschmann (*Der Andere Milton* (1920)), who consequently suggests that the poet's personality ought to be studied in the light of Adler's *Individualpsychologie* which, as is well known, exchanges the hegemony of the sexual impulses of Freudian psycho-analysis for that of the individual craving for power. Mutschmann also sheds much light on the relation between the power-complex, stoicism and 'satanism' in English Renaissance literature, Puritanism and, especially, in Milton (pp. 79 ff).

6. *Op. cit.*, pp. 81–3.

7. Words in roman type are for emphasis.

Zephon himself is fully conscious of his superior goodness, i.e., strength, and scorns Satan the '*wicked and thence weak*' (*ibid.* 856). Similarly

All wickedness is weakness.

S.A. 834

Adam (i.e., Milton himself) is scared to death at the power of female charm and beauty,[8] and no wonder Milton's better self, in this case the angel, answers with 'contracted brow'. Even Satan himself is overpowered;[9] in his own words:

Shee fair, divinely fair, fit Love for Gods,
Not terrible, though terrour be in Love
And beautie

ix. 489–91[10]

and similarly:

Yet beauty, though injurious, hath strange power.

S.A. 1003

This power-reaction to values is extremely significant, and very largely determines the atmosphere of the poem.

Milton's preoccupation with the ideas of kingdom, power and glory, has some interesting, more purely literary repercussions, apart from the more general question that Christian meekness and the power-complex seem hardly reconcilable.[11] The fact is that Milton, 'writing as a bitter anti-royalist drew heavily on the royalist literary tradition. A contradiction between the symbol and the idea was inevitable'.[12] But Milton does more than draw on a conventional symbolism. Royalty as the expression of majesty and power triumphant is something wherein he exults, wherein, *qua* poet, he lives and moves and has his being. There is practically no character in *Paradise Lost*, whether in heaven, in hell or on earth, who is not, at one time or another, called king or prince!

Activity is an expression of power and necessarily commands attention; and with the attention also a certain amount of sympathy, at least, if there is nothing to compensate for the inactivity on the other

8. *P.L.* viii. 546–59.

9. *P.L.* ix, ll. 457–66, obviously do not mean what Mr. Lewis reads into them. Satan is perplexed, dumbfounded, temporarily paralysed, as it were.

10. Words in roman type are for emphasis.

11. For this aspect of the matter see pp. 75–8.

12. Cf. M. M. Ross, *Milton's Royalism: A Study of the Conflict of Symbol and Idea in the Poems* (1943). Mr. Ross believes that Milton became aware of this contradiction and sought in his last poems to purify his idiom.

side. In an epic, potential, latent power is of little value; and it lies in the nature of Milton's fable that there is nobody to compete with Satan. Adam plays a passive role, and, as I have already pointed out, the expression 'domestick Adam' seems adequately to describe the nature of the 'power, rule, and dominion', which Milton wanted to bestow on him. The teeming activity of hell on the one hand, and the quietistic adoration and leisure in heaven and on earth on the other, are the true cause why the former is so impressive.

This goes so far that Mr. Hamilton[13] actually doubts whether the angels are really as happy. They are neither hungry nor overtasked, drink rubied nectar, and 'take recreation from somewhat shadowy tasks' in 'exercising heroic games'.[14]

For what is going on in heaven and Paradise is rather a sham activity. It lacks the element of risk and struggle, which is the decisive (and dramatically interesting) characteristic of human endeavour. Incidentally, in his attitude to activity, Milton is a classical exponent of the Renaissance tradition, for which action was all in all. Even a Milton cannot produce heroic effects without heroic action.[15] There is much truth in Mr. Wright's suggestion[16] that Adam's passivity, as a mere spectator to the depressing panorama of human misery in Books XI and XII, may be responsible for their comparative failure, rather than the 'Restoration disillusionment' or 'age and ill-health' assigned as causes by Dr. Tillyard and Mr. Lewis respectively. The hell of *Paradise Lost* has nothing to do with the traditional *inferno*. It reminds us rather of the headquarters of an underground movement, with Satan as the superior, fearless, and competent general. Except for the degradation passages, he is surrounded by an aura of majesty and power. I have already referred to the character of the similes employed by Milton to describe Satan and his partners. The various accounts of Satan's preparations to battle, fearless to the point of recklessness, even against heavy odds (unlike God and his Son, who only fight to parade their omnipotence), are really grand and inspiring, as, for instance, his encounter with Sin and Death and with Gabriel.[17]

That the basic human problem which is the subject-matter of *Paradise Lost*, must be considered and solved on the power-level, is suggested by Milton's delineation of Christ's character. Both Satan and the Son[18] are power-carrying figures, and Milton's 'desired end is an understanding

13. *Op. cit.*, p. 36.
14. *P.L.* iv. 551.
15. Cf. Tillyard, *op. cit.*, pp. 282–4, 290.
16. *Art. cit.*, p. 83.
17. *P.L.* ii. 706–23 and iv. 968–95.
18. Actually both are 'sons' in various gnostic sources. Cf. Jung: *Symbolik des Geistes* (1948), pp. 111–12, notes 128, 129 and 130, p. 252, note 60, p. 407, note 20.

of Christ as a figure of power not less but greater than military heroes and emperors'.[19]

Christ is conceived as the only power capable of conquering hell, both in their first battle,[20]

O're Shields and Helmes, and helmed heads he rode
Of Thrones and mighty Seraphim prostrate,

P.L. vi. 840–1

Yet half his strength he put not forth, but check'd
His Thunder in mid Volie, . . .

Ibid. 853–4

as well as in their last and final one:

For never but once more was either like
To meet so great a foe. . . .

Ibid. ii. 721–2

'Undoubtedly Satan is heroic and a great power . . . such heroism and power can only be overthrown . . . by a more deeply conceived heroism and a greater power',[21] i.e., the Messiah.

To grasp the full import of the power problem with Milton, it is necessary to go beyond the express data of the poems, and to state the issue in its widest theological significance. For power is one of the paramount factors in life, both as an insatiable craving and appetite in man, and as the decisive fact in human affairs.

It is from an awareness of the 'power' or 'energy' (*mana*, *orenda*, *wakonda*), present and active in the universe, that religion, or at least the 'dynamistic' religions arose. *Die primitiven Religionen in den verschiedensten Gebieten der Erde sind auf dieses Bild* [*der Energie*] *gegründet*, says Professor Jung,[22] and consequently rejects the idea of 'animism', as used by James and Frazer, for Lovejoy's more relevant term 'primitive energetics'. In fact primitive myths and rites are originally responses to this awareness, and attempts to express and handle this mysterious power.[23]

Scripture leaves no doubt that it considers power as an attribute, if not 'the attribute' of God. Indeed, He alone has power and every other power in heaven and on earth is derived from Him. This characteristic is not unique for power alone. Practically every positive aspect of life is conceived later along similar lines. Mere 'being' as such, as well as

19. G. Wilson Knight, *op. cit.*, p. 115.
20. *P.L.* vi. 710–18, 825–37. 21. G. Wilson Knight, *op. cit.*, p. 183.
22. *Ueber die Psychologie des Unbewussten* (5th ed., 1943), pp. 123–5.
23. See Harrison, *Themis*, Chap. 3. part., pp. 72–3 and Chap. 5.

the various modes of being, i.e., qualities and virtues, are God's; they come from Him, and to possess them is expressed as a sort of participation in Him, 'in whom we live and move and have our being'. (*Eph.* iv. 6, *Iohn*a xiv. 20–1, xvii. 21–3.) What is particularly insisted on in the passages referred to, is the participation in glory *through* that in active love. But all the other modes of life and being also are just so many other participations.

Life and history become a problem through the fact that there are so many uncoordinated participations, in other words, because in our 'fallen' world God's attributes are not equally, i.e., proportionally diffused and realized. Thence we meet goodness without power, and power without goodness. The conflict is, in principle, a familiar one, though in our world, where 'good and evil grow up together almost inseparably', the oppositions are never as absolute as they are in fairy tales. It is the challenge of 'authentic strength . . . matched against unrealized virtue'.[24] The hard truth is that 'goodness, not backed by authentic energy is of all things the most pitiful and even blasphemous for it makes game of God's most cherished purpose . . . humanity in whom goodness and power coexist'.[25] Goodness without power is more often hollow pharisaism, sloth, lack of virility and enterprising heroism, comfortably mistaken for virtue, submission to God's will and Christian martyrdom. Power, on the other hand, even without goodness, represents a real value, though usurping its God-given possibilities for ungodly purposes. We shall discuss at a later stage Milton's awareness of this 'dilemma of civilization', propounded to Adam by Michael,

> . . . *Those whom last thou sawst*
> *In Triumph and luxurious wealth, are they*
> *First seen in acts of prowess eminent*
> *And great exploits, but of true vertu void;*
> *Who having spilt much blood, and don much waste*
> *Subduing Nations, and achievd thereby*
> *Fame in the World, high titles, and rich prey,*
>
> *P.L.* xi. 787–93

particularly ll. 789–90

Power is thus the crucial test of the real and solid inner substance of goodness; the test that is to say, of whether it is a sham façade or a realization-in-power. 'Ethical superiority must not blind us to authentic power as arraigned against goodness-without-power, which is often verbose self-righteousness. Therefore the power thrust is a real chal-

24. G. Wilson Knight, *op. cit.*, p. 13. 25. *Ibid.*, p. 14.

lenge.'[26] As St. Paul has put it: '. . . the Kingdom of God is not in words, but in power'.[27] Consequently defeat through power-failure must be accepted as an implicit condemnation, and cannot be glossed over by the self-righteous weakling's pet consolation that he has been overcome 'by sheer brute force'. '. . . the established order, which is overthrown . . . falls through not being good enough; either not sufficiently powerful or not sufficiently elastic'.[28]

Of course this truth easily lends itself to misrepresentations by whoever *wants* to misunderstand. Probably this aspect of the matter has led Sir H. Grierson[29] to assert that Milton's doctrine is 'a dangerous one that might be used to justify Lenin or Mussolini or Hitler alike, the justification of success'. It may be worth while, by way of illustration, to follow for a moment Professor Grierson's method, and to try to clarify the issue by examples from modern history. We should then have to say that the policy of the western democracies which led up to the Second World War, was a glaring example of 'peaceful sloth', hiding behind some genuine values, but unable to meet the decisive test. The corresponding instance of value borne by authentic energy, was Gandhi's revival of the Indian doctrine of *satyagraha* and *ahimsa*, which to him was more in the nature of an ontological fact than a moral duty. In Gandhi's spiritual experience, truth, love, and non-resistance were no moral 'ideals' in our sense of the word, but ultimate goodness-equals-power facts. He believed in the efficacy of love above a machine-gun in precisely the same business-like and sober way, as we believe in the superiority of a machine-gun to a dagger, or of an atomic bomb to a machine-gun.

In Scripture the power-concept undergoes a considerable and highly interesting development which is very germane to our inquiry. Even as the God of the Old Testament does not allow his goodness, holiness and mercy to overshadow his (at times daemonic) power,[30] so his admonitions to his people always stress the connection between strength and goodness.[31] The doctrine is borne out by the interpretation of history as given in *Joshua*, *Samuel* and *Kings*, as well as by the prophetic speeches. God's people are given a religious task and a promise; but as for the latter, they have to fight it out. In the books of the Old Testament 'a small but virile nation is shown, subjecting its will-to-power to the service of some transcendent God, who demands

26. *Ibid.*, p. 147.
27. 1 *Cor.* iv. 20.
28. G. Wilson Knight, *op. cit.*, p. 39.
29. *Op. cit.*, p. 63.
30. Cf. Paul Volz, *Das Dämonische in Jahwe* (1924).
31. *Deut.* xxv. 18, xx. 1 ff., xxviii. 1–14, xxxiii. 29; *Lev.* xxxiii. 6–8.

. . . an ever more sensitive goodness'.[32] In the course of time a process of individuation set in, in which the divine love-mercy and daemonic-power aspects differentiated ever more sharply, and which finally culminated in a complete dissociation of the two elements in the Old Testament Apocrypha and in the New Testament. Part of what was formerly God is cast out; the devil becomes what psychologists call an autonomous complex[33] (*Revelation* 12, 9), and henceforward rules as the Prince of this World. On the other side God becomes the loving Father in a way which, according to Reinhold Niebuhr, makes the Christian conception of him 'more grandmotherly than fatherly'. The Kingdom can no longer be fought and striven for in an earthly effort. It can only be prayed, waited and suffered for. Christ, the Lamb of God, comes to stand exclusively for

Love without end, and without measure Greace,

whilst God's terror and awful power is no longer a source of direct and immediate experience.

Yet the ultimate unification of power with goodness, that is to say, the vision of God's holy power triumphant on earth as it is in heaven, is so imperative a need of the human soul, and consequently so deeply embedded in Scripture, that it cannot simply get lost. It insists and obtrudes itself because it is a basic psychic necessity. But as it has no longer any foothold in the realities of the New Testament and the later Old Testament, it gets associated exclusively with the end of time and the Last Judgement. In other words, *the solution of the power-problem turns eschatology*!

The relevance of this parallel from Jewish religious history to the understanding of Milton has also been noticed by Sir Herbert Grierson:[34] 'Milton's mind has passed through the cycle, which Dr. Charles describes in the progress of Jewish prophetic and apocalyptic literature, postponing to a remoter future, and ultimately to the coming of a new heaven and a new earth, the hopes for a Messianic kingdom.'

Many of the paradoxes already mentioned find their explanation in

32. G. Wilson Knight, *op. cit.*, p. 10. According to Professor Wilson Knight every great literature has the same end: 'The harmonising of virility and goodness [is] its ultimate purpose.'

33. The above is one of Miss Schärf's main conclusions in her detailed and penetrating study, 'Die Gestalt des Satan im Alten Testament' (in Jung: *Symbolik des Geistes* (1948), pp. 151–319). For a very short and very superficial outline of the development of Satan in the period under discussion, I refer to Edward Langton's *Satan*, pp. 9–14.

34. *Op. cit.*, p. 80.

this eschatological framework, described by Milton (*P.L.* iii. 311 ff.): meekness here and glorification in the hereafter, the last here being the first there, poverty on earth as laying up treasures in heaven and the like, are all images foreign, in that specific sense, to the earlier Old Testament. As far as we are concerned here, the most interesting consequence of this development is that the human craving for heroic action and noble struggle, for power-realization in the service of redemptive effort, has no correspondence in the God-Christ image. The only real, immediately accessible power-carrier is, at present, the Prince of this World, Satan. For 'where there is vigour, there is a tendency to overstep just bounds',[35] and Lucifer incarnates both that vigour and that tendency. The corollary is that every human effort and achievement, for every achievement is the result of effort and a manifestation of power, comes perilously near to the Satanic, and is in danger of condemnation. Pietism seems the word.

It is evident that the New Testament treatment of the problem raises some very grave questions, and it seems that the theologian Volz has voiced an important need when declaring: '*So ist der Gott des Alten Bundes nicht ein überwundener Gott. Ich möchte viel eher sagen, dieser Zug des alttestamentlichen Gottes und der alttestamentlichen Frömmigkeit den wir beschrieben haben, ist etwas was wir* zurückgewinnen *und bewusst behaupten müssen. Es ist schienbar etwas besonders Altertümliches am Alten Testament, dieses Dämonische in Gott*; *in Wirklichkeit aber ist es in aller Wandlung und Entwicklung, etwas Ursprüngliches und Ewiges.*'[36] It is surely not accidental that attempts to found God's Kingdom on earth always shows a strong return to the Old Testament. One of the greatest of these attempts, involving the use of military power, was the Commonwealth, to which Milton had devoted his life.

The split and conflict as regards the relation between power and goodness, inherent in the Christian scheme, is exemplarily illustrated by Milton, who mirrored it in his own nature. I believe this split to be

35. Already Masson had analysed 'activity' as the main element of Satan's character and as the cause of his fall.

36. Volz, *op. cit.*, p. 41. This is to revive the conviction of *Hebrews* x. 31: 'It is an awful thing to fall in the hands of the living God.' It is worthy of remark that whereas Volz wants to return to this attitude, Professor Dodd (*The Epistle of Paul to the Romans* (1932), p. 29) wants to get away from it. 'Paul, with a finer instinct [than the writer of Hebrews] sees that *the really awful thing is to fall out of His hands.*' Though ultimately agreeing to the italicized part of Professor Dodd's formulation, I cannot subscribe to it in its present context. His antithesis with *Hebrews* x. 31, shows that what he tries is less to really 'transcend' the daemonic aspect of God, than, on the contrary, the more modern escape of exonerating God from all demony by idealizing and moralizing him.

deeper and graver than is usually assumed. Even more, I believe it the one important split in Milton's personality, whereas all the others so much talked about are either non-existent or negligible. It is not that Milton's Puritanism was divided against itself in the sense that the ethical and religious elements in him, his 'hebraic righteousness' was at odds with his republican political passions,[37] nor, to quote a German scholar, that his art is formed by an amalgam of two conflicting character-traits: '*Die Gewalt des hinausstürmenden Titanen, der Schmerz und die bitterste Reuė sind in den Handlungen seiner Gedichte ausgegossen. Die Schönheit der klassischen Kunst hat seine Sinne gefangen wie die Leidenschaft seiner eigenen Brust es tat. Aber dagegen steht das Grübeln, der unerbittliche Ernst der Miltons Gedanken zum Himmel zwingt und sie nicht heimisch werden lässt auf dieser Erde, das starke Gefühl der sittlichen Pflicht*...[38] Mr. Hamilton seems to have fallen into the same error when judging Milton's 'vehement moral sense at odds with his poetic imagination'[39] and concluding that 'we see in *Paradise Lost* a notable division between Milton the sensuous and passionate, and Milton the Moralist'[40] and that 'The Satan, who dominates the scene is created by Milton the sensuous and passionate poet. The voice of opposition, in which the moralist speaks alone... sounds... weak.'[41]

This sounds all very beautiful, but it really means very little, and as far as it means anything, it is wrong. The truth rather is, as Professor Haller has pointed out, that Milton's Puritanism confirms rather than contradicts his poetry. 'The essence of his *biographia literaria* is that, when in the cultivation of his gifts he found his way to the poetry of the ancient world and the Renaissance, he found not distraction and escape from the Puritan urge to salvation and service, but the strongest possible confirmation'.[42] '... he never acknowledges the war between poetry and Puritanism, which may be after all nothing but the reflection of our own divided souls.'[43]

It seems to me that one-half of the really great conflict in Milton was that between his genuine New Testament Christianity and his equally

37. C. H. Herford, *Bulletin of the John Rylands Library*, viii, 223: 'Milton's Puritanism was divided against itself. If its ethical and religious element, the Hebraic passion for righteousness, made for the degradation and humiliation of Satan, the political passion of the republican involuntarily ennobled and glorified the assertor of liberty against the enthroned despot in heaven.' McLachlan (*op. cit.*, p. 21) still adds that 'this Puritan dichotomy escaped observation in the eighteenth century.'

38. Siebert, 'Untersuchungen über Miltons Kunst vom psychologischen Standpunktaus', *Anglia*, liv (1930), 82.

39. *Op. cit.*, p. 9. 40. *Ibid.*, p. 37. 41. *Ibid.*, p. 39.

42. Haller, *The Rise of Puritanism* (1938), pp. 306–307. 43. *Ibid.*, p. 289.

strong and genuine Old Testament character, which Ezra Pound so gracefully called 'his beastly Hebraism'.[44] When Professor Wilson Knight says[45] that Milton's disjointed work is an X-ray of his fractured period, one might add: and of his conflicting self. This is a usually neglected part of Milton's biography, but the discord can be traced from *Paradise Lost* through *Paradise Regained* to *Samson Agonistes*, as well as in his prose writings. From the many ecclesiastical pamphlets we know how thoroughly he detested power in the Church. The Church of Christ should neither employ power herself, nor ally herself to the powers that be. His break with Cromwell was over the absolute separation of Church from State. But one feels that what Milton really wants is true, authentic power, and that he senses the danger threatening the Church through false and inauthentic power. It is from this danger that he feels he must save the Church, lest her sense of real power corrupt, and she become 'an ass bestriding a lion'.[46] Yet the metaphor of the ass and the lion does not prevent us from finding in *Samson Agonistes*, which 'reflects Milton's own story as surely as the Tempest reflects Shakespeare's', his 'strongest revulsions projected into Dalila, his deepest longings into the divinely ordained strength of Samson',[47] who is Milton's final attempt to fuse virility with goodness and to conceive of strength as God-given, yet proudly physical.

To understand fully the evolution of Milton's attitude towards power, heroic energy, and enterprising action, we should have to consider *Paradise Regained* more closely. But this may be done more conveniently when we come to consider the place accorded by Milton to civilization and culture as the specific expression of human activity and achievement.[48] It may suffice here to state the problem in the pregnant formulations of Professor Wilson Knight. '*Paradise Lost* is a poem of unresolved discords, with its central conflict lingering after the supposed resolution has been asserted. There is, certainly, a specious schematic unity in terms of divine over-lordship and reason, but the Satanic energies, though clamped down, are not stilled . . . underneath great energies seethe' . . .[49] 'Milton was a fighter, his every accent exults in power; but he was a Christian. In what sense can power be Christian?'[50] Jesus is a heroic, royal figure of Samson-like strength, and when we read *Paradise Regained*, iii. 71 ff., we must wonder: 'Is not military prowess a primary Miltonic joy? Is it not the Messiah's

44. In an essay written in 1918 and reprinted in *Make it Now* (1934). See Logan Pearsall Smith, *Milton and his Modern Critics* (1940), pp. 17–18.
45. Wilson Knight, *op. cit.*, p. 17.
46. *Reason of Church Government.*
47. Wilson Knight, *op. cit.*, pp. 83–5.
48. Cf. p. 82.
49. Wilson Knight, *op. cit.*, p. 121.
50. *Ibid.*, p. 102.

chief glory in *Paradise Lost*? . . . Is not all Milton's work crammed to overloading with images of kingly might and God himself in *Paradise Lost* conceived on the direct analogy of a human tyrant . . .? The answer is obvious: that with God things are different. But the doubt lingers.'[51] In *Paradise Regained* Jesus appears as a pacifist, though far from mild.[52] Satan's attack on the pacifist position agrees with our feeling that Christ, as an earthly, not merely spiritual king, has 'to assume flesh and blood, to come down from his lonely pinnacle of irrelevant righteousness and reign . . .'[53] 'But Satan's eminently reasonable arguments . . . are totally unsuccessful. He is somewhat baffled; so are we and so I think was Milton,' says Wilson Knight.[54]

This perplexity is natural as long as we are at a loss to grasp the relation between the ass and the lion, between 'Christ the Lamb' and 'Christ the Tiger'. Our instinctive feeling is that if the Messiah cared to show his power right now, the world would be better off. We are apt to cling to this belief, in spite of Jesus' contemptuous dismissal of it,

Plausible to the world, to me worth naught.

P.R. iii. 393

In this respect Milton's interpretation of the Temptation of Christ in a way anticipates Dostoievski's Great Inquisitor. In accordance therewith Professor Wilson Knight believes that critics are usually silent about *Paradise Lost*, vi. 824 ff. because 'a truly power-impregnated righteousness is as yet alien to our thinking, and all but outside our vision'.[55] Consequently, 'the poem is an honest facing of an all but insoluble difficulty. . . . The poem offers no synthesis.'[56]

What must we conclude from all this? In the first place that there is a necessary ambiguity about the character of Satan. Beginning as the unproblematical protagonist of what was perhaps the most popular fable (a fable which begins before the Creation and which ends with Doomsday), he loses his simplicity through his relation with the great universal drama, which is the drama of the will of God omnipotent, striving to be done on earth as it is in heaven. That the Son of God and heir to his Kingdom has taught the world to pray for its coming,[57] otherwise leaving the world to its own devices instead of actively interfering, only tends to complicate matters further.

51. Wilson Knight, *op. cit.*, pp. 102–3, 107. 52. *Ibid.*, p. 102.
53. *Ibid.*, pp. 108–9. 54. *Ibid.*, p. 111. 55. *Ibid.*, p. 162. 56. *Ibid.*, p. 115.
57. And Milton could do so very fervently! Cf. his *Animadversions* '. . . Come forth out of thy royal chambers, O Prince of all Kings of the earth, put on the *visible* [!] robes of thy imperial majesty, take up that unlimited sceptre which thy Almighty father hath bequeathed thee'.

Secondly Satan, as rebel against a rather passive God's immutable decrees, becomes the symbol of the power-carrier who strains every muscle, nerve and fibre against a supreme and unrelenting, and *ipso facto* cold and hostile fate. This practically makes him symbolic of the human condition in general, of

. . . the dread strife
Of poor humanity's afflicted will,
Struggling in vain with ruthless destiny.

(Who is not reminded here of Prometheus!) For we too are up against a hostile, cold and hard world, and so, from a different point of view, is even Christ. What perplexes us is that Christ's manner of dealing with the situation is so strange and inexplicable, so unlike our own and Satan's, which appears to us as the only sensible one. Satan (and in a way we too) thus usurps and arrogates to himself that which really belongs to God and His Son, that to which Christ has laid claim, but which he refuses to wield—until the fullness of time will have come. We would prefer active battle, the risk and flux of war on the pattern of early Old Testament history, to the eschatological faith which we can mainly serve by standing and waiting.

Some critics may identify the Satan of *Paradise Lost* with King Charles, but he certainly *also* is 'Cromwell casting an "experienced eye" over his ironside warriors. The comparison . . . complicates our understanding: for Satan is not merely dramatically impressive—his case is pretty nearly Milton's'.[58] And therefore, thirdly, 'through Satan, Milton might be said to express and half-condemn his own impatient demand for the perfect Christian order'.[59]

So far we have endeavoured to trace some correspondences between the delineation of Milton's Satan and some of the most fundamental and urgent facts of human psychic reality, particularly as expressed in Scripture. Within the Christian frame, Milton's Satan figure responds to a considerable degree to our inner self and to some of its gravest and noblest images and aspirations. After all that has been said so far, it will be clear how it has come about that these aspirations of our struggling self present themselves in the figure of him who fell through inordinate pride, and who since then roams the earth as Satan, Fiend and Devil. But if the earth and the fullness thereof, the world and they that dwell therein, are no longer the Lord's, but are ruled by their new Prince, our next concern must be to examine the possible attitudes to such a world, and in particular the attitude of the Christian that was Milton.

58. G. Wilson Knight, *op. cit.*, p. 127. To this must be added that God's reign in *Paradise Lost* is one of Law, whilst the Satanic order is one of free consent. (*Ibid.*, p. 134.)

59. *Ibid.*, p. 113.

Chapter Five

SIN IS BEHOVELY

Sin is Behovely, and
All shall be well, and
All manner of thing shall be well.

T. S. ELIOT, *Four Quartets*

BEFORE beginning our analysis of Milton's texts, it may be advisable to summarize and restate the conclusions of the preceding chapters, mainly in order to get the proper setting for their interpretation.

We have found in *hubris* a psychic necessity on the way of individuation and differentiation towards higher levels of consciousness.[1] In its Promethean form this means that human life involves trespasses and real violations of the divine, albeit static order, and the inevitability of doing wrong in a very objective sense of the word. To all this is added a new and specific kind of suffering. Even for Aeschylos, let alone for Hesiod, Prometheus is in trespass. He may be a criminal, or a tragic sinner, but sinner he is, and not merely the hero of a righteous war of liberation against cruel tyrants, as a certain school would have it. Since Zeus' order is that of a static cosmos, every human aspiration and effort is a revolt.

As we have seen the Christian order,[2] particularly as mirrored in

1. pp. 29 ff.

2. The world is the devil's, who is its Prince. (*John* xii. 31, xiv. 30.) The rapprochement between the Promethean and the luciferic worlds as outlined in this and the previous chapter, is actually based on a still more basic rapprochement which I have failed so far to mention, and which ought to have had its place in Chapters 2 and 3. It is the problem of the fall of Lucifer as a hybridic phenomenon, corresponding to a decisive step in the evolution of consciousness. (Cf. also C. G. Jung, *Die Beziehungen zwischen dem Ich und dem Unbewussten* (4th ed., 1945), p. 61, note 1.) I have desisted from treating the subject here, because it is too profound and subtle to admit of a summary and perfunctory mention, and lack of space makes it impossible to give it its full due. All I can do therefore is to refer the reader to the literature on the subject, but first and foremost to C. G. Jung's volume *Symbolik des Geistes* (e.g., pp. 112, 140–8, 439 ff. and Miss Schärf's essay, *ibid.*, pp. 274, 291 ff.). Cf. also *infra* 33, note 18, and p. 64. Speculations on the ambivalent and 'luciferic' character of Satan are, of course, not modern. They belong to the stock-in-trade of all gnostic and heretical sects and systems, ancient and modern. But as one can safely say that

Milton's work, is in many ways similar. God is leading history his own way, whilst man's activity as such is revolt and sin. The fact that, theologically speaking, God's plans and providence, unlike those of Zeus, are supposed to be ultimately beneficial to mankind, does not really change the immediate situation. The only real difference is that in the Christian picture we have the creator-creature dependence,[3] which makes sin the more heinous and literally rebellious.

The Lucifer-Prometheus myth thus becomes capable of different developments. The one may consist in a deliberate choice of Satan (Blake, Byron) either through accepting his vitality whilst ignoring the significance of his evil, or by going to the length of accepting even evil itself as a mark of vitality and for its sake (Nietzsche). Another possibility is to substitute Prometheus for Satan, i.e., to find a symbolic expression for human existence which does not involve the full horror and demony of the traditional Christian devil (Shelley). The third possibility would be to follow the first group in their identification of the Satanic and the Promethean, but to draw the opposite conclusion: to condemn them both, and implicitly all human achievement.

That the latter was the way of historical Christianity, or to put it more accurately, that Christianity never succeeded in steering clear of this danger, needs no proof here.[4] What matters here, is that this same attitude is strongly discernible in Milton, in spite of his 'materialism', Hebraism, and Renaissance-activism, which manifested themselves

---

so far all attempts to link Milton with these movements and systems have failed, I feel justified in neglecting this *tiefenpsychologische* aspect of the matter, and to concentrate more on the Promethean and cultural one. For this at least we are not dependent on mystical speculations, but can draw in profusion on Miltonic texts.

3. Hence Lucifer's fall begins with the heresy of regarding himself as eternal and self-created (*P.L.* v. 853–66). Similarly Avitus, *De Spirit. Hist. Gest.*, Bk. II. *de originale peccato*, 38 ff. writes:

> *Angelus hic dudum fuerat, sed crimine postquam*
> *Succensus proprio tumidos exarsit in ausus,*
> *Se semet fecisse putans, suus ipse creator*
> *Ut fuerit, rabido concepit corde furorem*
> *Auctoremque negans: 'Divinum consequar, inquit,*
> *Nomen et aeternam ponam super aethera sedem*
> *Excelso similis summis nec viribus inpar.*

It is strange to note that this remarkable parallel has escaped the attention of all those who have compared Avitus with Milton, often with a view to establishing the former as a 'source' of *P.L.* Cf. Guizot, *Histoire de la Civilisation en France*, (6th ed., 1857), ii. 59–69; M. J.-J. Ampère, *Histoire Littéraire de la France avant le 12e siècle* (1839), pp. 197–9; S. Gamber, *Le Livre de la Genèse dans la Poésie Latine au 5e siècle* (1899), p. 253.

4. Cf. pp. 35, 64.

inter alia in his full and whole-hearted co-operation in the Commonwealth. The passages where Milton testifies to his awareness of the possibility of a divinely inspired civilization have already been quoted.[5] But they sound very weak and tame when compared with his exposition of the Promethean theory of civilization as expounded in Mammon's splendid speech

> . . . *but rather seek*
> *Our own good from our selves, and from our own*
> *Live to our selves, though in this vast recess,*
> *Free, and to none accountable, preferring*
> *Hard liberty before the easie yoke*
> *Of servile Pomp. Our greatness will appeer*
> *Then most conspicuous, when great things of small,*
> *Useful of hurtful, prosperous of adverse*
> *We can create, and in what place so e're*
> *Thrive under evil, and work ease out of pain*
> *Through labour and indurance.*
>
> *P.L.* ii. 252–62

The first six lines have a strong Graeco-Roman flavour, whilst the last six describe a civilization inspired by Satan. Similarly Michael blasts Adam's happy optimism at his vision (Book XI, 556–92) which

> . . . *attach'd the heart*
> *Of* Adam, *soon enclin'd to admit delight,*
> *The bent of Nature*
>
> *Ibid.* 595–7

with a stern Puritan

> *Judg not what is best*
> *By pleasure, though to Nature seeming meet,*
> *Created, as thou art, to nobler end*
> *Holie and pure, conformitie divine.*
>
> *Ibid.* 603–6

But Milton gives us more details, ranging from the most material to the most spiritual aspects of culture. These are scattered throughout *Paradise Lost*, but the two main texts are the description of the fallen angels' activities in hell, and the visions plus commentaries granted to Adam in the last books of the poem. Thus, to begin somewhere, the first organized activity of the Satanic party is mining from a volcano in hell:

5. p. 64.

There stood a Hill not far whose griesly top
Belch'd fire and rowling smoak; the rest entire
Shon with a glossie scurff, undoubted sign
That in his womb was hid metallic Ore,
The work of Sulphur.

P.L. i. 670–4

in fact this art *par excellence* of the *homo faber* is of hellish origin:

. . . by him first
Men also, and by his suggestion taught,
Ransack'd the Center, and with impious hands
Rifl'd the bowels of thir mother Earth
For Treasures better hid.

Ibid. 684–8

Newton's note, quoted from Warburton, should be mentioned here, as illustrating how deep this association is apparently engrained in popular imagination. According to him:

'Milton alludes in a beautiful manner to a superstitious opinion, generally believed among the miners: That there are a sort of Devils which converse much in minerals, where they are frequently seen to busy and employ themselves in all the operations of the workmen; they will dig, cleanse, melt, and separate the metals. See G. Agricola, *De Animant. Subterraneis. . . .*'

The precise historical account is told in Adam's vision.

In other part stood one who at the Forge
Labouring, two massie clods of Iron and Brass
Had melted . . .
. . . the liquid Ore he dreind
Into fit moulds prepar'd; from which he formd
First his own Tooles; then, what might else be wrought
Fusil or grav'n in mettle.

P.L. xi. 564–73

One should keep in mind here the difference between Cain's toiling and iron-founding posterity,[6] and the idyllic, extremely righteous, but rather unproductive Sons of Seth.[7] The subject of mining of course also includes heavy industries in general, and in particular the manufacture of arms. The inventions of iron-mining and artillery are actually

6. On the scriptural basis of these Miltonic verses and their Promethean affinities, see pp. 34 ff.

7. *P.L.* xi. 573–80.

identified, when Satan breaks his great news after their first lost battle.[8] Satan here takes the place of Mammon of Book I[9] and of Hephaistos,[10] the iron-forger and smith who too fell from heaven, limping since then like the popular Christian devil.[11] Milton still adds a beautiful aperçu about technical inventions which has been repeated in numberless variations,

Th'invention all admir'd, and each, how hee
To be th'inventor miss'd, so easie it seemd
Once found, which yet unfound most would have thought
Impossible

P.L. vi. 498–501

and forecasts the baneful application of this invention:

. . . *yet haply of the Race*
In future dayes, if Malice should abound,
Some one intent on mischief, or inspir'd
With dev'lish machination might devise
Like instrument to plague the Sons of men
For sin, on warr and mutual slaughter bent.

Ibid. 501–6

Fascinating is the description of the angelic war-effort. For unlike the philosophers and theologians so heartily loathed by Milton,

None arguing stood, innumerable hands
Were ready, in a moment up they turnd
Wide the Celestial soile, and saw beneath
Th'originals of Nature in thir crude
Conception; Sulphurous and Nitrous Foame
They found, they mingl'd, and with suttle Art,
Concocted and adusted they reduc'd
To blackest grain, and into store convey'd:
Part hidd'n veins diggd up (nor hath this Earth
Entrails unlike) of Mineral and Stone,
Whereof to found thir Engins and thir Balls
Of missive ruin; part incentive reed
Provide, pernicious with one touch to fire.

Ibid. vi. 508–20

8. *P.L.* vi. 472–91. 9. ll. 684–8. 10. *Ibid.*, 739 ff.

11. *Le diable boiteux*, *Hinkebein*, already appears in the Anglo-Saxon *Andreas*, 1173, as *helle-hinca*. In connection with Hephaistos, it may be added that also the smith of northern legend, Weland, is lamed in his legs, but does manage to construct wings for himself!

Much has been said about the invention and use of artillery by the fallen angels. Mitford,[12] though doubting whether Milton really knew the many Italian plays on his subject named since Voltaire, nevertheless found this coincidence with Valvasone's *Angeleida* particularly 'worthy of remark', but Newton, Masson and others have already shown that the idea occurs in many preceding poets, including Ariosto and Spenser. What I believe to be far more significant is the profoundly typical interpretation Milton gives this incident in his further account of the battle. For after a first *échec* by the Satanic broadsides,

> *. . . the excellence, the power*
> *Which God hath in his mighty Angels plac'd*
>
> *Ibid.* 637–8

again assert themselvs and

> *Thir Arms away they threw, and to the Hills*
>
> . . . . .
>
> *Light as the Lightning glimps they ran, they flew,*
> *From thir foundations loosning to and fro*
> *They pluckt the seated Hills with all thir load,*
> *Rocks, Waters, Woods, and by the shaggie tops*
> *Up lifting bore them in thir hands*
>
> *Ibid.* 639 ff.

and throw them on the rebellious host. Addison, who greatly admired the 'bold thought' of ascribing the heavy artillery to the devils, qualified the angels' tearing up of hills as 'not so daring', since already Ovid's giants had been throwing Ossa upon Olympus and Pelion upon Ossa. The real point of the incident lies, of course, in the equation of goodness with nature (i.e., fighting with hills) on the one hand, and of the satanic power-craving and explosive *hubris* with technique and machinery on the other. The gunpowder is Satan's own invention and his Salmoneus-like bid to out-thunder Jove. This aspect of the matter is expressly and repeatedly stated:

> *. . . they shall fear we have disarmd*
> *The Thunderer of his only dreaded bolt.*
>
> *Ibid.* 490–1

> *eternal might*
> *To match with thir inventions they presum'd*
> *So easie, and of his Thunder made a scorn,*
>
> *Ibid.* 630–2

12. Advertisement, the Aldine edition of *Milton's Poetical Works* (1832), vol. i, pp. x–xi, note 6.

The obvious association with Prometheus Milton has incidentally expressed in one of his youthful 'conceits', the last of the Latin gunpowder verses, *In Inventorem Bombardae*:

> *Japetionidem laudavit caeca vetustas,*
> *Qui tulit aethereum solis ab axe facem;*
> *At mihi major erit, qui lurida creditur arma,*
> *Et trifidum fulmen surripuisse Jovi.*

It almost goes without saying that Milton responds to his own Arthurian inclinations by letting the devils indulge in chivalric exercises,[13] even as he rewarded music for its ministry and solace by giving it a place in hell, where devils move

> *In perfect* Phalanx *to the* Dorian *mood*
> *Of Flutes and soft Recorders;*
>
> *P.L.* i. 550–1

and

> *Retreated in a silent valley, sing*
> *With notes Angelical to many a Harp*
> . . . . .
> *Thir Song was partial, but the harmony*
> . . . . .
> *Suspended Hell, and took with ravishment*
> *The thronging audience.*
>
> *Ibid.* ii. 547 ff.

The indictment of music is repeated in the vision of Adam,[14] to which is joined that of poetry and dancing.[15] Apparently not even cattle-breeding is exempt from this Puritan nihilism,[16] much more so then the more adventurous and active temperament of the Elizabethan and Milton's own age, where new discoveries and exploits acted as a continual ferment inviting bold extension of former limits,

> *Another part in Squadrons and gross Bands,*
> *On bold adventure to discover wide*
> *That dismal world, if any Clime perhaps*
> *Might yield them easier habitation, bend*
> *Four ways thir flying March.*
>
> *Ibid.* 570–4[17]

13. *P.L.* ii. 528–38.
14. *P.L.* xi. 558–63.
15. *P.L.* xi. 583–4.
16. *P.L.* xi. 556–8.
17. Mention must be made in this connection of Mutschmann's thesis (in 'Studies concerning the origin of P.L.' in *Acta et Commentationes B*, v (Dorpat, 1924)) that Satan is 'identified with the early English explorers of the North-East passage, Sir H. Willoughby and R. Chancellor'. Cf. the quotation from Tillyard, p. 103.

Those devils who engaged in neither warlike feats nor music, sat apart on a hill retired, in sweet discourse and elevate thoughts,

. . . and reason'd high
Of Providence, Foreknowledge, Will and Fate,
Fixt Fate, free will, foreknowledg absolute,
And found no end, in wandring mazes lost.
Of good and evil much they argu'd then,
Of happiness and final misery,
Passion and Apathie, and glory and shame,

Ibid., 558–64

discussing, in fact, the agenda of the Westminster Assembly. The hierarchy of values, i.e., of Milton's aversions, must be noted too. The description of hell progresses from chivalry to music, and thence to philosophy. Hume noted[18] that 'our poet so justly prefers discourse to the highest harmony, that he has seated his reasoning angels on a hill as high and elevated as their thoughts, leaving the songsters in their humble valley'.

Newton commented on the 'elevated discourse' as follows:[19]

'Good and evil and de fin. bon. et mal. etc., were . . . the subjects . . . among the philosophers and sophists of old, as providence, free will, etc., were among the school-men and divines of later times, especially upon the introduction of the free notions of Arminius upon these subjects: and our author shows herein what an opinion he had of all books and learning of this kind.'

Adam is instructed by Raphael himself as to the range he should permit his reasoning faculty, and is taught to live

The easiest way, nor with perplexing thoughts
To interrupt the sweet of Life, from which
God hath bid dwell farr off all anxious cares,
And not molest us, unless we our selves
Seek them with wandring thoughts, and notions vain.
But apt the Mind or Fancie is to roave
Uncheckt, and of her roaving is no end;
Till warn'd, or by experience taught, she learne,
That not to know at large of things remote
From use, obscure and suttle, but to know
That which before us lies in daily life,
Is the prime Wisdom, what is more, is fume,
Or emptiness, or fond impertinence,

18. *Ad. P.L.* ii. 550–60. 19. *Ad.* l. 565.

And renders us in things that most concerne
Unpractis'd, unprepar'd, and still to seek.
Therefore from this high pitch let us descend
A lower flight, and speak of things at hand.

P.L. viii. 183–99

A generation later Pope was to advise:

Trace science, then, with modesty thy guide,
First strip off all her equipage of pride.

Essay on Man, ii. 43–4

What Raphael, i.e., Milton, indoctrinates, is the scientific attitude of paradise which Erasmus had already described in his *Moriae Encomium*: 'In the first golden age of the world there was no sort of learning.... They were not so presumptuous as to dive into the depths of Nature, to labour for the solving all phenomena in astronomy, or to wreck their brains in the splitting of entities ... judging it to be a crime for any man to aim at what is put beyond the reach of his shallow comprehension.'

That this sort of 'practical wisdom' can be as wrongheaded as the other is subtle and unreal, Milton has demonstrated in his *Treatise* and pamphlets. Masson has tried to neutralize the effect of this diatribe against learning by pointing to 'Milton's enthusiastic outburst on the pleasures of scientific research and speculation in the third of his *Prolusiones Oratoriae*, and also his advocacy of Physical Science in his *Tract on Education*', whereas Newton thinks the passage 'socratic'.

Milton's attitude towards stoicism has already been discussed.[20] The stoic complaint 'from the famous distich of Euripides, which Brutus used when he slew himself'[21] is voiced by the fallen angels, lamenting

... that Fate
Free Vertue should enthrall to Force or Chance.

P.L. ii. 550–1

whilst Milton at the same time allows his other feelings to peep out in such lines as:

Eve, *thy contempt of life and pleasure seems*
To argue in thee somthing more sublime
And excellent then what thy minde contemnes;

P.L. x. 1013–15

Yet he who reigns within himself, and rules
Passions, Desires, and Fears, is more a King;
Which every wise and vertuous man attains;
And who attains not, ill aspires to rule

20. pp. 39–44.

21. Newton, *ad loc.*

Cities of men, or head-strong Multitudes,
Subject himself to Anarchy within,
Or lawless passions in him which he serves.

P.R. ii. 466–72

What wise and valiant man would seek to free
These thus degenerate, by themselves enslav'd,
Or could of inward slaves make outward free?

Ibid., iv. 143–5

One may well ask who is speaking here if not the pagan philosopher! But the fact that Satan's followers build, dig for gold, make music and philosophize, means that man's total culture is condemned. The attempt to explain these facts away by distinguishing between culture created for godly and for depraved ends[22] is too naïve, and altogether ignores the inner dynamism of the verse.

Whereas in *Paradise Lost* Milton's condemnation of civilization is rather piecemeal and indirect, in *Paradise Regained* the attack is delivered in its most general, explicit and radical form. For here all the values and achievements of 'the world' are presented one by one by Satan, and contemptuously dismissed by Jesus. The 'temptation' of heroism Jesus had experienced early within himself:

. . . *victorious deeds*
Flam'd in my heart, heroic acts, one while
To rescue Israel *from the* Roman *yoke* . . . etc.

P.R. i. 215–17

whereas Satan confronts him with the various means of active intervention in the affairs of our world. Riches:

. . . *thy heart is set on high designs,*
High actions; but wherewith to be atchiev'd?
Great acts require great means of enterprise,

. . . . .

Therefore, if at great things thou wouldst arrive
Get Riches first, get Wealth, and Treasure heap

Ibid., ii. 410–12, 426–7

power:

. . . *with what ease*

. . . . .

22. 'The diversions of the fallen angels . . . are every way suitable to beings who had nothing left them but strength and knowledge misapplied. Such are their contentions at the race, etc. . . . Their music is employed in celebrating their own criminal exploits. . . .' (Addison.)

Might'st thou expel this monster from his Throne
Now made a stye, and in his place ascending
A victor people free from servile yoke?
And with my help thou may'st; to me the power
Is given, and by that right I give it thee.

Ibid., iv. 97–104

and wisdom.[23] Jesus' 'Puritan' rejection of all culture is notorious.[24] As has already been said, this expostulation is all the more remarkable in view of the whole tenor of Jesus in *Paradise Regained*, his thoroughly Greek haughtiness and stoic morals. Still more remarkable is that, in spite of his theoretical condemnation of this culture, Milton could never forbear expressing his admiration and reverence for its great exponents. Leaving aside Galileo and turning to antiquity, we find the old Roman heroes compared without qualms to Gideon and Jephthah;[25] mainly, it should be admitted, because they too were poor! Socrates is placed right next to Job himself,[26] and Milton supports his anti-Calvinist thesis that 'some remnants of the divine image still exist in us' by an appeal to 'the wisdom and holiness of many of the heathen, manifested both in words and deeds'.[27] Even in his worst moments Jesus has to make exception for those parts of pagan philosophy

. . . where moral vertue is express't
By light of Nature not in all quite lost.

P.R. iv. 351–2

But riches are peremptorily refused

Extol not Riches then, the toyl of Fools,
The wise mans cumbrance if not snare,

Ibid., ii. 453–4

and so is power:

Much ostentation vain of fleshly arm,
And fragile arms, much instrument of war
Long in preparing, soon to nothing brought,
Before mine eyes thou hast set; and in my ear
Vented much policy, and projects deep
Of enemies, of aids, battels and leagues,
Plausible to the world, to me worth naught.

Ibid., iii. 387–93

23. *P.R.* iv. 221–84. See following note.

24. *P.R.* iv. 285–364. This highly important passage is unfortunately too long to be quoted here.

25. *P.R.* ii. 439–47.

26. *P.R.* iii. 95–9.

27. *Treatise*, Bk. I, Chap. 12. Col. ed., vol. xv, p. 209.

The real issue here is that of an active political realism versus a half moral, half religious quietism. Satan's arguments

... thy Kingdom though foretold
By Prophet or by Angel, unless thou
Endeavour, as thy Father David *did,*
Thou never shalt obtain; prediction still
In all things, and all men, supposes means,
Without means us'd, what it predicts revokes.

P.R. iii. 351–6

each act is rightliest done,
Not when it must, but when it may be best,

Ibid., iv. 475–6

summed up by Jesus:

Means I must use thou say'st, prediction else
Will unpredict ...

Ibid., iii. 394–5

as well as his general attack on the pacifist position, are eminently reasonable, whereas Jesus' answers are everywhere open to objections. Neither the contention that he

May also in this poverty as soon
Accomplish what they did, perhaps and more

Ibid., ii. 451–2

nor the other, that wealth without virtue, valour and wisdom is

... impotent
To gain dominion or to keep it gain'd

Ibid., 433–4

explains why he who has succeeded in attaining all these virtues, governing his inner man and 'reigning within himself' as a 'true' king, should not also assume might and riches, wield power and

... rule
Cities of men, or head-strong Multitudes.[28]

It is useless to point to the development of Milton's political and psychological theories: that only those who have established the kingdom of reason within themselves could hope to improve the world, and that the failure to see this was the true cause of the failure of the revolution. This may suffice as an account of Milton's theoretical evolution from the Commonwealth via *Paradise Lost* and *Paradise Regained* to *Samson Agonistes*, where the hero, after confessing his fault and gloriously

28. See p. 78.

overcoming temptation, can finally act again, albeit in an assertion of self-destructive heroism. But it is certainly inadequate as an account of the dynamism of the verse, whose tension, power and *élan* strain in another direction. In a significant 'besides' Milton betrays to what extent all his talk about 'first rule yourselves, then rule the world' as well as Jesus' declaration

. . . who best
Can suffer, best can do; best reign, who first
Well hath obey'd; just tryal e're I merit
My exaltation without change or end

P.R. iii. 194–7

are but eyewash:

Besides to give a Kingdom hath been thought
Greater and nobler done, and to lay down
Far more magnanimous, then to assume.

Ibid., ii. 481–3

The hopelessness of the dilemma is set forth by Satan in his temptation-programme:

. . . with manlier objects we must try
His constancy, with such as have more shew
Of worth, of honour, glory, and popular praise;
Rocks whereon greatest men have oftest wreck'd;
Or that which only seems to satisfie
Lawful desire of Nature, not beyond;

Ibid., 225–30

where the crux is in the last two lines. The minimum aspirations of man, his 'lawful desires', what are they? and when and how is their satisfaction permitted? The trouble is that even if we were converted to Milton's theories, his verse would contradict them, particularly when we match its dynamic sweep against its intellectual contents and the unconvincing background of eschatological procrastination in which the latter is set. Jesus' answers[29] may possibly be true. Here theologians and philosophers are free to take sides. But the literary critic is equally free to point out that the passages in question show more haughty pedantry and inconclusive prevarication than genuine messianic *élan* and expectation.

In the alternatives offered by Jesus, Milton gives himself away badly, and plainly shows how little there was in him of the true religious mystic and how much of the Greek idealist. For the solution proferred by Jesus is persuasion. He holds it

29. *P.R.* iii. 182–7, 396–402; iv. 146–53.

. . . more humane, more heavenly first
By winning words to conquer willing hearts,
And make perswasion do the work of fear;

P.R. i. 221–3

and regards himself as called

. . . to guide Nations in the way of truth
By saving Doctrine, and from errour lead
To know

Ibid., ii. 473–5

as if the ministry of Christ consisted in his 'teaching'! Milton may have had an inkling of the power and reality of authentic spiritual superiority;[30] that power which all mystics know, and which St. Paul meant when he spoke about conquering evil through good or about God's weakness and foolishness confounding our strength and wisdom. It is a faith such as is expressed in the legend of St. Francis and the wolf, and such as our own age has witnessed in the life of Gandhi. It is the invisible power of the spirit which 'from heart to heart is stealing' and thence to the head. It travels from the heart and the reins to the brain, whereas idealists first of all want to put ideas into the head, and very often never come to think of the heart and the reins at all. It is not Christ who wants to 'convince' or 'pursuade' people, but Plato who tries to found his ideal kingdom by indoctrinating young tyrants. This distinction is not accidental. It even has its precise counterpart in the Biblical and Greek cosmogonies. For the Jews the world exists because the *creator spiritus* evoked creative response with his creative word: 'And God said, Let there be light: and there was light'[31] whereas for the Greek mind: 'intelligence has mastered blind necessity [*ananke*)] because she succeeded in persuading [*peithein*] her to provide for the better for most things. And it is thus, through blind necessity giving way to the persuasion [*peitho*] of intelligence, that from the beginning the world has formed itself.[32]

30. 'The kingly function of Christ is that whereby being made King by God the Father, he governs and preserves, chiefly by an inward law and spiritual power, the Church which he has purchased for himself, and conquers and subdues its enemies . . . "chiefly by an inward law". . . . Herein it is that the pre-eminent excellency of Christ's kingdom over all others as well as the divine principles on which it is founded, are manifested; inasmuch as he governs . . . not by force and fleshly weapons but by what the world esteems the weakest of all instruments'. (*Treatise*, Book I, Chap. 15. Col. ed., vol. xv, pp. 297–301.)

31. *Gen.* i. 3.

32. Plato, *Timaios*, 48 A. In other words, the cosmic order consists in God 'persuading' chaos to function in an orderly way! See F. M. Cornford, *Plato's Cosmology*, (1948), p. 35 ff.

It is therefore difficult not to agree with Professor Wilson Knight, when he calls the figure of Christ in *Paradise Regained* 'cold, negative, almost nihilistic to culture' and compares it to Cromwell.[33] This basically unbiblical nihilism is a typical fruit of late and post-Old Testament mythology in interpenetration with the pagan world, and should be regarded as a consequence of the full development of the Satan-image and the appearance therein of Promethean characteristics. I would not belittle the connection of the texts of *Paradise Lost* Book, XI referred to, with *Genesis* iv. 17–24, where we are told that Cain and his seed were the originators of city-building, cattle-breeding, music and iron-forging. But it is here as with so many other Biblical myths and motives, which can be discovered by a close analysis, but which remain practically irrelevant and without importance, leading a rather shadowy sham-existence, until at a given moment they suddenly start to life again and even come into a central position. Such is, e.g., the existence of demons, not excluded by the Old Testament, but almost completely forgotten, until in the apocryphal and New Testament period they reawaken, and we get a full-blown demonology. Such is the story of the fall and original sin, and such is also the myth of civilization as diabolic. What Milton has to say on the subject belongs less to *Genesis* iv, than to the apocryphal *Book of Enoch*[34] which repeatedly rehearses the story of the fall of angels, elaborating the bare account of *Genesis* iv. with much fantastic detail, and in particular giving long lists of the names of the fallen angels and of their ministrations to man. Chapter 8 tells us that:

'Azazel taught man to make swords, and knives, and shields, and breastplates, and made known to them the metals . . ., and the art of working them, and bracelets, and ornaments, and the use of antimony, and the beautifying of the eyelids, and all kinds of costly stones. . . . Semjaza taught enchantments, and root-cuttings, Armaros the resolving of enchantments, Baraqijal [taught] astrology, Kokabel the constellations, Ezeqeel the knowledge of the clouds. . . .'[35]

Similarly we read in Chapter 69:[36]

'The name of the first Jeqon: that is, the one who led astray [all] the sons of God, and brought them down to the earth, and led them astray through the daughters of men. And the second was named Asbeel: he imparted to the holy sons of God evil counsel, and led them astray so that they defiled their bodies with the daughters of men. And the third was named Gadreel: he it is who showed the children of men

33. *Op. cit.*, p. 115.
34. See Charles, *The Apocrypha and Pseudepigrapha of the Old Testament*, vol. ii.
35. *Ibid.*, p. 192.
36. *Ibid.*, pp. 233–4.

all the blows of death, and he led astray Eve, and showed [the weapons of death to the sons of men] the shield and the coat of mail, and the sword for battle, and all the weapons of death to the children of men. . . . And the fourth was named Penemue: he taught the children of men the bitter and the sweet, and he taught them all the secrets of their wisdom. And he instructed mankind in writing with ink and paper, and thereby sinned from eternity to eternity and until this day. For men were not created for such a purpose. . . .'

This list is practically identical with that which Prometheus gives of his services to mankind. For originally, man

Who first, with eyes to see, did see in vain,
With ears to hear, did hear not, but as shapes
Figured in dreams throughout their mortal span
Confounded all things, knew not how to raise
Brick-woven walls sun-warmed, nor build in wood,
But had their dwelling like the restless ant,
In sunless nooks of subterranean caves.
No token sure they had of winter's cold,
No herald of the flowery spring or season
Of ripening fruit, but laboured without wit
In all their works, till I revealed the obscure
Risings and settings of the stars of heaven.
Yea, and the art of number, arch-device,
I founded, and the craft of written words,
The world's recorder, mother of the Muse.
I first subdued the wild beasts of the field
To slave in pack and harness and relieve
The mortal labourer of his heaviest toil,
And yoked in chariots, quick to serve the rein,
The horse, prosperity's proud ornament.
And none but I devised the mariner's car;
On hempen wing roaming the trackless ocean.

. . . . .

Of all the greatest, if a man fell sick,
There was no remedy, nor shredded herb
Nor draught to drink nor ointment, and in default
Of physic their flesh withered, until I
Revealed the blends of gentle medicines
Wherewith they arm themselves against disease.
And many ways of prophecy I ordered,
And first interpreted what must come of dreams

In waking hours, and the obscure import
Of wayside signs and voices I defined,
And taught them to discern the various flight
Of taloned birds, which of them favourable
And which of ill foreboding, and the ways
Of life by each pursued, their mating-seasons,
Their hatreds and their loves one for another;
The entrails too, of what texture and hue
They must appear to please the sight of heaven;
The dappled figure of the gall and liver,
The thigh-bone wrapt in fat and the long chine
I burnt and led man to the riddling art
Of divination; and augury by fire,
For long in darkness hid, I brought to light.
Such help I gave, and more—beneath the earth,
The buried benefits of humanity,
Iron and bronze, silver and gold, who else
Can claim that he revealed to man but I?
None, I know well, unless an idle braggart.
In these few words learn briefly my whole tale;
Prometheus founded all the arts of man.

Prom. 463–84, 494–522

Of the hell of *Paradise Lost* Professor Wilson Knight has said 'that it is peopled by beings of tragic wisdom and masterful resolve'[37] in short, by Prometheuses. But precisely because of that, his other dictum, that in Satan Milton expresses and half-condemns his own impatient demand for a perfect Christian order,[38] is inadequate. What Milton 'half-condemns' is much more than that. It is everything Prometheus stands for, in a conception which regards every human assertion and progress as a trespass, committed under the high patronage of the father of all self-assertion and hybridic trespass: Lucifer, alias Satan, alias the devil, alias the Prince of *this* World. As he is the sole power-carrier in our present universe,[39] every progress and activity is asso-

37. *Op. cit.*, p. 135.
38. Cf. p. 79.
39. Cf. p. 75. That this attitude is somewhat archetypal is proved by other parallels. E.g., the Germanic Loki, originally a fire-elf and as such typically ambivalent, once helpful then harmful, but finally becoming the cause of the death of Baldr (the god of light), and the centre of a number of hellish beings (*Hel*, the *Mithgarth* serpent, the *Fenriswolf*). For a recent account see Frank Stanton Cawley, 'The Figure of Loki in Germanic Mythology', *Harvard Theological Review*, xxxii (1939), 309–26.

ciated with him and dissociated from God, and is, consequently, in need of salvation.

Here, I think, is the root of the trouble with *Paradise Lost.* Milton's treatment of Satan and of the problem of history and civilization may go against the grain of more modern-minded Christians, and they would be loath to admit that the late Archbishop's strictures on the poem[40] as a failure, really imply the relative failure of Christianity. We have a Zeus-like God, a Son who as yet refuses to wield power, and a humanity which, because it is created in a Creator-God's own image, is brimful of enterprise and creative energy. In the prevailing psychic constellation however this energy is 'bedevilled' and sacrificed to the *hubris* fear-complex. Lucifer, not being worshipped, is thus condemned, and with him Prometheus with whom he now is associated.

What expedients are left open in this situation?

40. W. Temple, *op. cit.*, p. 8. Cf. p. 39.

Chapter Six

TO OBEY IS BEST

ONE of the results of an analysis of *Paradise Lost* and *Paradise Regained* is the discovery that the ambivalence of Satan is matched by a similar ambivalence in the delineation of Christ's character. The full revelation, in an eschatological frame, of his power-contents, coalesces with the final defeat of Satan and the assumption, by Christ, of his power attributes. It is in that sense that Professor Wilson Knight feels that Christ in *Paradise Regained* 'is not the ideal discussion partner with Satan', because ultimately he himself is 'a heroic, royal figure of Samson-like strength',[1] and the desired end is 'an understanding of Christ as a figure of power not less, but greater than military heroes and emperors'.[2] In fact Michael has to cut a rather poor figure in his encounter with Satan, because 'nothing less than the Messiah can prove victor over his heroic virility',[3] and we are made to feel that even if Satan has 'revolutionary ardour, democratic reason and barbaric virility' and a host of other fine qualities, yet the Messiah is 'something higher and greater. . . . Undoubtedly Satan is heroic and a great power . . . such heroism and power can only be overthrown by a more deeply conceived heroism and a greater power.'[4]

Inversely we might say that Christ and Satan are two differentiated sides of a more primitive divine image, which must, and this has to-day assumed the rank of a question of life and death, be reintegrated again on a new level. When Jung speaks of '*jene Doppelfigur . . . welche hinter der Gestalt des Christus und des Diabolus zu stehen scheint*,' to wit the mysterious Lucifer,[5] and refers to *Revelation* xxii. 16, where Jesus says of himself: '*Ego sum radix et genus David, stella splendida et matutina*,' we might add a phrase from the *Exultet* of Easter Eve, the splendid *Praeconium Paschale*, which expressly calls Jesus the Lucifer: *Flammas eius* (of the paschal candle) *lucifer matutinus inveniat, ille inquam Lucifer*

1. *Op. cit.*, p. 103. 2. *Ibid.*, p. 115. 3. *Ibid.*, p. 150.
4. *Ibid.*, p. 183. 5. *Symbolik des Geistes*, p. 112.

qui nescit occasum. The brilliant and paradoxical formulation fits well into that unique and splendid piece of liturgy, which also contains the famous and equally paradoxical *O Felix Culpa.*[6]

The obvious corollary would be that in the meantime Satan performs an important function in the cosmic household. I do not refer at present to the mystical and gnostic idea of God himself needing, as it were, Satan in order to realize Himself—an idea on which the analytical psychology of Jung is throwing new light to-day—and which is already implicitly contained not only in the Biblical Satan, but also in the Prometheus figure of Aeschylos, who through his rebellion has an important share in the change that takes place in Zeus and so in his relation to the world.[7] I would limit myself at present to the conventional theory of evil performing its function by ultimately serving the good. As Goethe's Mephistopheles describes himself:

> . . . *Ein Teil von jener Kraft*
> *die stets das Böse will und stets das Gute schafft.*

In another, still more poignant saying, Goethe compares the world to a great organ 'played by God, whilst the devil is treading the bellows'. This brings us into the neighbourhood of Blake's conception of Satan as mere passion and energy, unformed, unharnessed, 'uncircumcised' as it were. At any rate the doctrine of evil as subservient to God's purposes, notwithstanding its factual opposition to His will, is an orthodox and almost trite commonplace. It can be traced in medieval literature, and is repeatedly stated by Milton.[9] The relation of the *Paradise Lost* passages to the medieval paradox of the Fortunate Fall has been discussed by Professor Lovejoy.[8] What seems of far-reaching consequence is that this idea has largely determined the traditional attitude of the Church to the 'world' and matters 'temporal'. But this view of the devil's 'not ignoble' function is a highly problematical one. It is tenable only so long as its acceptance is, as it were, unconscious

6. My reason for not expatiating at length on the theme of the 'Fortunate Fall' and the paradox of evil is already stated by implication in note 2 to Chapter 5. It goes without saying that the spiritual climate wherein the *Felix Culpa* idea could grow, is the indispensable background and presupposition for much of what is said in these chapters. But their sole object is to investigate the specifically Promethean side of the picture.

7. On the theory of a progressive Zeus see Harrison, *Themis*, and the literature given by Thomson, *op. cit.*, p. 12, note 4. See also Rex Warner's introduction to his translation of the *Prometheus Bound.*

8. *P.L.* vii. 187 ff; 613 ff; xii. 469–78; 585–7.

9. 'Milton and the Paradox of the Fortunate Fall', *E.L.H.*, iv (1937), now also accessible as Chap. 14 of his volume *Essays in the History of Ideas* (Baltimore, 1948). Cf. also Taylor, *Milton's use of Du Bartas* (1933), p. 22.

and realized willy-nilly by the mere fact of existing in this world and participating in its life. It is, at its best, the description of a retrospective attitude. Professor Wilson Knight's conclusion: '. . . We can feel Milton's Satan, himself ancestor to great things in Goethe, Byron and Shelley, as present humanity, whose final warring calls down Messiah. Satan has his function, and not an ignoble one' asks for an important reservation, because its application is limited to the analysis of past events only. When having to chose in a concrete situation, this beautiful paradox is obviously more disturbing and useless than helpful. With every growth of consciousness the problem becomes more intolerable because the contents of *good* and *evil* become less and less unequivocal whilst at the same time man is confronted with the increasingly clear and unequivocal choice: Satan or Christ—unless he is prepared to face the difficult task apparently posed by our present state of consciousness, that of a radical psychological revision of the values of good and evil.

It is therefore not surprising to find the devil-image reappearing in varying forms and guises with every crisis of consciousness, that is to say with every new assertion of man, manifesting itself as a step forwards. The image was pretty prominent at the birth of Christianity, and again with the Renaissance (Marlowe) and the Reformation (Luther).[10] We find a corresponding image active again in our time, mainly in connection with the quaternity-archetype.[11] The satanic power-surge so characteristic of our time runs riot in the enormous inflation of some of the worst elements of the collective *psyche* and in the identification by the masses of archetypes with their national or other monster-organizations.

In order to obviate the charge of partiality liable to be brought against the preceding account, it may be useful to restate the same in non-mythological and more rationalist language. The best witness here is certainly Bertrand Russell, whom nobody will suspect of a particular weakness for the tenets of analytical psychology and from whose *History of Western Philosophy* I would therefore quote:[12]

'The Greeks, with their dread of *hubris* . . . carefully avoided what would have seemed to them insolence towards the universe. The Middle Ages carried submission much further: humility towards God was the Christian's first duty. Initiative was cramped by this attitude and great

10. It is also usually overlooked that witchcraft trials, etc., were unknown in the 'Dark Ages'. They flourished between the sixteenth and seventeenth centuries, and particularly in the latter!

11. Cf., e.g., Jung, *Psychologie und Religion* (1947); pp. 66–9, 94 ff.

12. pp. 855–6.

originality was scarcely possible. The Renaissance restored human pride, but carried it to the point where it led to anarchy and disaster. Its work was largely undone by the Reformation and the Counter-reformation. But modern technique, while not altogether favourable to the lordly individual of the Renaissance, has revived the sense of the collective power of human communities. Man, formerly too humble, begins to think of himself as almost a God.'

Russell then goes on to speak of the intoxication of power which he regards as the greatest danger of our time and which is a direct consequence of the successive removal of the traditional checks upon human pride. The diagnosis is the same as has been made by psychologists in their analysis of current social symbols and of the dreams of neurotic patients.

Particularly the Marlovian conflict is of interest here, because Faustus introduces the modern assertion of man as a power-and-sensuality craving sponsored by the devil. One might add perhaps that the preponderance of the diabolic or Promethean elements in these images largely depends on the corresponding God-image, that is to say on whether the latter is represented with the anthropomorphic Biblical character, or closer to the Greek concept of fate and a cosmic order. Whereas Shelley's idealist atheism can as a consequence idealize the Satanic myth into the purely Promethean, the courage (and perversity) to be of the devil's party increases with the rush towards our modern crisis of consciousness (Blake, Byron, Nietzsche[13]) and is to a great extent an attempt to justify this dynamism. The trouble obviously does not lie with antinomianism as such, but with a psychic constellation which feels uneasy at this dynamism and which wants a justification of it. Professor Wilson Knight has summed up the problem in the following words: 'Mystical philosophers from Luther to Nietzsche have reacted violently and with superb energy away from the static and conceptualized culture of the European tradition: in them burn the Renaissance fires from which the upspring of German militarism and will to domination is not finally to be dissociated. Perhaps the best of all definitions of the Renaissance and the Medieval-Christian in clashing discord is offered by Marlowe's plays, which point unmistakably to Nazi Germany. Tamburlaine . . . Dr. Faustus deliberately presents the Renaissance power-quest—scientific, aesthetic and militaristic—with Faust himself reborn to new youth, in vivid conflict with medieval

13. Whose *Zarathustra* is almost contemporary with Spitteler's *Prometheus and Epimetheus* (1882), to which it bears a striking resemblance. On Goethe's Faust, Spitteler's Prometheus and Nietzsche's Zarathustra see C. G. Jung, *Psychologische Typen*, Chap. 5.

Christianity, rising to a shattering conclusion in which Christ's victory functions in the verse precisely as does Messiah's onset in *Paradise Lost*. The Germanic source of the Faust-legend is significant. The Jew of Malta. . . . The Marlovian conflict is . . . closely Miltonic'.[14]

To this dilemma, we must conclude, Milton has borne witness with all his poetic power. To the dichotomy of European consciousness equally deriving from Palestine and from Greece, Milton has given 'a local habitation and a name', whilst at the same time he has valiantly striven with himself to arrive at a solution. This striving found expression in an increasingly rigorous judgement on the world, and a continual hardening of attitude towards its achievements and values. His verse and diction become more harsh and austere, corresponding to his own 'slowly hardening intolerance'.[15] His recourse to classical mythology becomes rarer, until it ceases completely.[16] Yet I think the account Mr. Harding gives of this evolution to be slightly misleading. '. . . as the poet grew older he seems to have become more and more sceptical, herein reflecting the increasing rationalism of the seventeenth century. Finally, in *Paradise Lost* we encounter the curious situation where Milton may adorn a mythological allusion with some of his most magnificent poetry, and then, in the same breath as it were, may often proceed to denounce it as pagan fiction. . . But in the end the victory of rationalism was complete. The negative evidence of *Paradise Regained* and *Samson Agonistes* strongly implies that there came a time when he could no longer see any common ground of truth between classical mythology and Christian teaching. . . .'[17] I do not believe that 'increasing rationalism', at least in the ordinary sense of the expression, is the right word here, and the evidence from *Paradise Regained*, iv. 334 ff. is more than negative. It was not the victory of rationalism that was complete, but that of 'Sion' over 'Babylon', and that of a Puritanism, which did not shrink from appreciating Greek poetry as a mere imitation (and a bad one at that[18]) of Scripture. Of Milton's philosophy of history enough has been said already. The digest of his experience is summed up by Adam (*P.L.* xii. 561–73) and is confirmed by Michael,

This having learnt, thou hast attained the summe
Of wisdome; hope no higher, though all the Starrs
Thou knewst by name, and all th'ethereal Powers,
All secrets of the deep, all Natures works,

14. *Op. cit.*, p. 142.

15. Cf. Rajan's essay: 'Simple, Sensuous and Passionate', *R.E.S.*, xxi (1945), 300.

16. Cf. C. G. Osgood, *op. cit.*, xlvi–l; D. Bush, *op. cit.*, pp. 270–7; D. P. Harding, *op. cit.*, pp. 93–9.

17. *Op. cit.*, pp. 98–9.

18. *P.R.* iv. 338–9 ff.

Or works of God in Heav'n, Air, Earth, or Sea,
And all the riches of this World enjoydst,
And all the rule, one Empire; onely add
Deeds to thy knowledge answerable, add Faith,
Add Vertue, Patience, Temperance, add Love,
By name to come call'd Charitie, the soul
Of all the rest. . . .

P.L. xii. 575–85

These last words of Michael show the Christian attitude, or at least the Miltonic version of it, in its relatively most amiable and active light. Yet, on the whole, the general impression of hostility towards the world remains unrelieved even by the indication of a turn to another direction, discernible in *Samson Agonistes* and the last pamphlets. 'Acceptance', 'obedience', 'calm submission' are the words with which Professor Sewell[19] qualifies the period of *Paradise Regained* and *Samson Agonistes* in contrast with the 'doubts and spiritual conflicts' out of which *Paradise Lost* and the *Treatise* were born. One may disagree with many of Professor Sewell's interpretations and conclusions, but the epithets chosen are certainly the right ones.

These conclusions do not differ very much from those reached, in different ways, by Dr. Tillyard:[20]

'You cannot ignore him [Milton], any more than you can ignore Alexander the Great, or Cromwell, or Napoleon. He is too extraordinary a person to shut out from our notice; and he is perhaps the only man of his type, who has translated his mental urge into literature and not into action. I do not mean that he is a mere Tamberlane. His was no uncontrolled lust for mere conquest. Rather he typifies the controlled energies of the great explorers and inventors. He stands thus as a perpetual monument of the pioneering spirit in man, a spirit which may have destroyed much as well as created, have caused misery as well as happiness, but to which human civilization is largely indebted and which we cannot condemn unless we condemn civilization itself.'

What I would add to Dr. Tillyard's appraisal is the other half to his incomplete picture: that Milton, in fact, also condemned civilization; that he was highly distrustful of our exploring and inventive energies; and that he also stands as a perpetual monument of the spirit of cultural ascetism and negation.

No, Milton certainly is no antinomian. But in his poetry he is a curious and significant exponent of a critical feature of our civilization. He presents the conflicting elements not in compromise or synthesis,

19. *A Study of Milton's Christian Doctrine* (1939). 20. *Op. cit.*, p. 368.

but in unrelieved tension and active dialectics, lived at both poles with a remarkable intensity. He showed himself a Greek in both his Platonicism and *hubris*, and in his sense of their wrongness; and a Hebrew in his acceptance of the world and the senses, in the consciousness of his calling as a child of God, but also in his fear of the temptations of this earth.[21] Equally fearing the Scylla of sensuality and the Charybdis of pride, he was a typical—and great—European and Christian, who sought his God amid these tensions and tried to serve him in a world which he denounced and which at the same time he affirmed with all its glories. In this situation he had to make his Satan a Prometheus, and his Prometheus a Satan. Milton's Satan is great, and exhibits so many positive qualities because he has absorbed Promethean elements; and Prometheus is condemned because he is seen in the devil. This, it would seem, is one of the reasons which to us make *Paradise Lost* a failure.

But it is more than the failure of a poem only.

21. It is necessary to insist on the point, that by Hebraic and Greek I understand two basic, though highly different, sorts of *prise de conscience*, attitude, structures of experience, or whatever name we choose to give it. This is too often overlooked in discussions on Milton. So quite recently Mr. E. I. Watkin has been severely taken to task by Mrs. Margaret Bottral ('The Baroque Element in Milton', in *English Miscellany*, i (Rome, 1950), 35) for having said that 'Milton was too classical and too Hebraic to be called baroque'. For this he is now chided by Mrs. Bottral. 'One might begin by enquiring how a poet can be simultaneously too classical and too hebraic' (I hope to have shown in the present study that he can). 'Presumably Milton's moral fervour is felt to be hebraic, and his manner of writing latinized. . . . He discerns in Milton a temperamental inclination to Judaism, rather than to Catholicism, together with a certain coldness and hardness (this is where classical comes in). . . .'

I do not know Mr. Watkin's *Catholic Art and Culture* (1947), and cannot therefore judge whether Mrs. Bottral's account and criticism does justice to his intentions. But in this particular her criticism is certainly off the mark. The pagan world was not without its own 'moral fervour', and Milton's classicism is a matter also of psychic attitude, temperament, and sensibility, and not only a manner of writing.

APPENDICES

APPENDIX A

From William Blake, *The Marriage of Heaven and Hell:*

From these contraries spring what the religious call Good & Evil. Good is the passive that obeys Reason. Evil is the active springing from Energy.
Good is Heaven. Evil is Hell.

The Voice of the Devil

(Errors) (2) That Energy call'd Evil is alone from the Body, & that Reason call'd good, is alone from the Soul.
(3) That God will Torment Man in Eternity for following his energies.

(true) (2) Energy is the only life, & is from the Body; & Reason is the bound or outward circumference of Energy
(3) Energy is Eternal Delight.

Those who restrain desire, do so because theirs is weak enough to be restrained; and the restrainer or reason usurps its place & governs the unwilling. And being restrain'd, it by degrees becomes passive, till it is only the shadow of desire. The history of this is written in Paradise Lost, and the Governor or Reason is call'd Messiah. And the original Archangel, or possessor of the command of the heavenly host, is call'd the Devil or Satan, & his children are call'd Sin and Death.

But in the Book of Job, Milton's Messiah is called Satan.
For this history has been adopted by both parties.
It indeed appear'd to Reason as if Desire was cast out; but the Devil's account is that the Messiah fell, and formed a heaven of what he stole from the Abyss.
This is shown in the Gospel, where he prays to the Father to send the comforter, or Desire, that Reason may have Ideas to build on; the Jehovah of the Bible being no other than he who dwells in flaming fire.

Know that after Christ's death he became Jehovah.
But in Milton, the Father is Destiny, the Son a Ratio of the five senses, & the Holy-ghost vacuum!

Note: The reason Milton wrote in fetters when he wrote of Angels & Good, & at liberty when of Devils & Hell, is because he was a true poet & of the Devil's party without knowing it.

It is almost unnecessary to point out how much of the argument of the preceding study is anticipated in this quotation. What is actually needed is a 'translation' of Blake's intuitions (and errors!) into modern psychological language, together with a minute exegesis and an analytical commentary. As lack of space forbids such an undertaking here, I shall limit myself to a few remarks and pointers.

In the first place it appears that Blake is clearly aware of the problem of the ambivalence of the power and energy factor, and of the fact that in actual religious (read Christian) development, this factor has been 'bedevilled' and all but equated with evil (ll. 5–7). Blake moreover rightly feels that the conventional scheme of moral restraint and rational self-government comes dangerously near to complete passivity and sterility (ll. 15–16).

The passage implies a strong sense of the original vital unity of life (l. 10). *Energy* is Blake's word for Schopenhauer's *Wille* and our more modern *Life Force*, *élan vital*, etc., conceived not as an abstraction, but as the thrill of the fullness of life (ll. 10–12). With the appearance of Reason a counter-principle is introduced, which makes life a more differentiated complex. Reason, the secondary product of evolution, promptly usurps government and purports to legislate (ll. 14–15), the whole process being somewhat comparable to the growth of patriarchy gradually supplanting matrilinear society. Even so Blake feels that Reason is at its best but a formal principle which must draw for its life on Energy (ll. 10–11). Had he lived to-day, Blake would probably have said that the unconscious is the source of all psychic energy. The contents of 'consciousness' or 'reason' are supplied by the unconscious; they have 'flowed over' as it were. Blake's energy should perhaps not be equated solely with what Jung calls the *libido*, but also with the unconscious which contains the *libido*.

Blake's intuition of this differentiation ending in complete dissociation is of extraordinary brilliance. Dissociation of the elements of a complex whole is, of course, the expression used by a neutral observer, by the 'third party' as it were. To those who are bound up with one of the two sides, the fact that the original wholeness and unity is broken invariably means that the 'other' side has been cast out. (Incidentally 'the other side' is the technical term of the Kabbalah for Evil!) With a view to the original and undifferentiated God-image (ll. 26–9) it is equally legitimate to say that the devil has been cast out, as it is to affirm that the Angels have fallen (ll. 23–4). It is not always easy to distinguish between God and the Devil; 'and no marvel, for Satan himself is transformed into an angel of light' (2 *Cor.* xi. 14). As a matter of fact the unconscious can be constellated as God, viz., an angel of light or as the devil, according as it functions as a source of light and guidance to higher levels, or as the threat to swallow and submerge again whatever consciousness has been attained. This again depends on the strength, integrity and humility which consciousness has achieved.

From the point of view of the emergence of consciousness and *ratio* from the depths of the unconscious, Blake's formulation that the Messiah formed a heaven of what he stole from the abyss is sheer genius. After all, every inch of 'psychic territory' occupied by consciousness is conquered from the unconscious and thus is literally heaven stolen from the abyss! But as long as we are without objective and absolute standards, the same story can in fact be adopted by both parties (l. 22), although the telling differs in perspective. The total frame of the story remains the same; only the directions of the movements change—relative to the observer's position.

Blake's capital error consisted in his failure to see that nature quite objectively involves a genuine higher and lower. The 'higher' cannot exist without the 'lower', nor consciousness without the unconscious; but this fact does not invalidate the distinctive hierarchy. In his legitimate fight for the rights of the unconscious, Blake erred on its side, even as those against whom he championed its cause erred on the other. This is exactly the situation discussed in Chapter 2.

The 'error' (ll. 8–9) that God would torment man in all eternity for following his energies is obviously more than an error. It is man's consciousness of punishment laid up for him if he refuses to move to the higher levels to which he is called (or impelled) and chooses instead to remain in or to return to the motherly womb, the sea and fen of the unconscious. Apparently Blake thought himself immune against the complementary danger of aspiring too high: *hubris*. On the contrary, he brazenly prefers the abyss to heaven. But by flouting the other danger, he actually vitiated his own purpose: life untrammelled—because existence without limits is impossible and unthinkable. We here touch the relation of Blake to the castration-complex. His praise of virility and abhorrence of 'Goodness' and 'Reason' (equated by him with impotence) simply land him in the 'lower' or 'matriarchal' castration. It was not without profound reason that the priests and priestesses of the fertility-divinities of antiquity were virgins and prostitutes, sodomites and eunuchs.

It is interesting to note how Blake brushed by the solution, obviously unable to see its import because of the peculiar twist in his vision. His idea of reason as 'the bound or outward circumference of energy' (l. 11) should have carried the implication that a complex life, bi-polar as it were, and wavering between the attraction of the conscious and that of the unconscious, resolves itself into the problem of temperance and of the right limits. Circumcision is the Biblical answer to Blake's pseudo-alternative of boundless energy and impotence. (Cf. German *Be-schneiden* and *Ver-schneiden*.)

In his partiality Blake is the victim of a long religious and philosophical tradition which had succeeded in so abstracting and rationalizing the human soul, dissociating and severing it from its unconscious matrix and soil, that it could be identified with a divine or nearly divine intelligence and ratio. This one-sided abstraction was consequently regarded as *the* good and as the ultimate value. Blake's great error was to identify it also with the Messiah who is, in reality, the heroic re-conqueror of unity who finally overcomes man's existential duality. But although Blake went too far in his necessary reaction, and went definitely wrong in his disregard for the *coincidentia oppositorum*-function of the victorious Messiah, he yet was perfectly right in his description of the actual course of development of these collective representations, and of the actual function of these images in the conventional Christian scheme. The intuition that Milton's poetry reflected the strain and tension between these two poles, and the uneasy conscience at the bottom of our civilization, is Blake's great contribution to Miltonic criticism. I hope to have proved in the preceding chapters that Milton has in fact emasculated his Messianism by unconsciously proceeding from the same assumptions as Blake: that energy and creative vitality are Promethean and thus devilish, whilst Christ is Reason and his lesson is passivity, obedience and self-restraint.

APPENDIX B

Angels Celestial and Infernal

From Newton's Index of Similes

ANGELS CELESTIAL

Subject	*Image*
Spears of guardians of Paradise	ears of corn, ripe for reaping (*P.L.* iv. 980).
their march against Satan's army	that of the birds of Paradise receiving their names from Adam (vi. 72).
their hallelujahs	the sound of seas (x. 642).
appointed to expel Adam and Eve	a double Janus (xi. 128).
their eyes	those of Argus (xi. 129).
their appearance	angels in Mahanaim and to those in Dothan (xi. 213–16).
their motion	an evening mist (xii. 628).

ANGELS FALLEN

Subject	*Image*
	autumnal leaves (i. 302).
	floating sea-sedge after storm (304).
rousing at Satan's command	sentinels waking from sleep on duty (331)
imbattling against celestial angels	Egyptian plague of locusts (338)
	the irruptions of the northern barbarians (351).
their disposition to engage	that of the heroes of antiquity (549).
with them	the greatest armies pigmies (573).
themselves	oaks and pines blasted (612).
their searching for materials for Pandemonium	pioneers intrenching (675).
their manner of raising Pandemonium	the wind of an organ (705).
their assembling	bees and fairies (768 and 781).

their rising from Council	thunder far off (ii. 476).
their pleasure on the result	evening sun after foul day (488).
their various pursuits	Olympic or Pythian games (530).
	phenomena of armies in the clouds (533).
	Hercules on Oeta (543).

SATAN

Subject	*Image*
	Briaerus, Typhon, Leviathan (i. 199, 201).
	sun rising in mist (594).
	longest train of a comet (ii. 707).
	Mount Teneriff or Atlas (iv. 985).
his shield	the moon (i. 284).
his spear	a mast (292).
his standard	a meteor (337).
his ascent to hell-gates	a fleet in the offing (ii. 636).
his meeting with Death	two thunder clouds (714).
his flight to court of Chaos	a griffin's in the wilderness (943).
recoiling under Michael's blow	a mountain sinking by an earthquake (vi. 193).

It is true Satan also is a weather-beaten vessel (ii. 1043), a wolf preying on a fold (iv. 183), a thief breaking in at a house-top (iv. 188), a vulture seeking his prey (iii. 431) and even a toad.[1]

In contrast to Satan, Michael, when expelling Adam and Eve from Paradise, is merely like a man in a military vest (xi. 239). This combat with Satan is compared to two planets rushing on each other (vi. 310).

This selection speaks for itself. It seems as if Milton has bestowed all his poetic genius on the infernal party. There is nothing in the poem to balance the profusion of splendid descriptions and powerful similes lavished on Satan and his crew, or to make up for the stepmotherly niggardliness with which the good angels are treated. A poet who is all on the 'right' side would have been more careful in his distribution of impressive epithets!

1. That the form of a toad is one of the devil's favourites guises, is an old and highly orthodox doctrine. Already Pope Gregory IX knew all about it. (Cf. his bull *Vox in Rama*, of June 13, 1233, text in Ripoll: Bullar. ord.praed. Vol. I. No. 81.)

QUOTATIONS AND ABBREVIATIONS

Milton quotations have been made as a rule from the Columbia Edition. The Aeschylos quotations and translations are taken from *Aeschylus: The Prometheus Bound*, edited with Introduction, Commentary and Translation by George Thomson, Cambridge, 1932.

The titles of Miltonic works are usually given in full, except for *P.L.* = *Paradise Lost*, *P.R.* = *Paradise Regained*, *S.A.* = *Samson Agonistes*, and *De Doctrina Christiana* which is referred to as *Treatise*.

The abbreviation *Prom.* refers to the *Prometheus Bound* or *Prometheus Desmotes* of Aeschylos.

The abbreviations of Biblical books are the usual ones: e.g., OT = Old Testament, NT = New Testament, *Gen.* = *Genesis*, *Exod.* = *Exodus*, etc.

Harv. Theol. Rev.	=	*Harvard Theological Review.*
M.L.N.	=	*Modern Language Notes.*
R.E.S.	=	*Review of English Studies.*

BIBLIOGRAPHY

BODKIN, MAUD: *Archetypal Patterns in Poetry*. 1934.

BUSH, DOUGLAS: *Mythology and the Renaissance Tradition in English Poetry*. 1932.

CHARLES, R. H.: *The Apocryphe and Pseudepigrapha of the Old Testament*. 1913.

CRAWLEY, FRANK STANTON: 'The Figure of Loki in Germanic Mythology'. *Harv. Theol. Rev.* xxii. 1939.

CECIL, LORD DAVID: *Introduction to the Oxford Book of Christian Verse*. 1940.

EMPSON, W.: *Some Versions of Pastoral*. 1935.

FROMM, ERICH: *The Fear of Freedom*. 1945.

GREEN, CLARENCE C.: 'The Paradox of the Fall in Paradise Lost'. *M.L.N.* liii. 1938.

GRIERSON, HERBERT J. C.: Art. 'Vondel' in *Hasting's Encyclopedia of Religion and Ethics*.

Cross-currents in English Literature of the Seventeenth Century. 1929.

Milton and Wordsworth. 1937.

HADHAM, JOHN: *God and Human Progress*. 1944.

HALLER, WILLIAM: *The Rise of Puritanism*. 1938.

HAMILTON, G. R.: *Hero or Fool? A Study of Milton's Satan*. 1944.

HANFORD, J. H.: *A Milton Handbook*. 1927.

HARDING, DAVIS P.: *Milton and the Renaissance Ovid*. 1946.

HARRISON, JANE: *Themis*. 2nd ed. 1927.

HEINEMANN, K.: *Die tragischen Gestalten der Griechen in der Weltliteratur*. 1920.

JUNG, C. G.: *Psychologische Typen*. 2nd ed. 1925.

Wandlungen und Symbole der Libido. 3rd ed. 1938.

'Psychologische Aspekte des Mutterarchetypus', in *Eranos-Jahrbuch*. 1938.

Uber die Psychologie des Unbewussten. 5th ed. 1943.

Die Beziehungen zwischen dem Ich und dem Unbewussten. 4th ed. 1945.

Psychologie und Religion. 1947.

Symboloik des Geistes. Studien über psychische Phänomenologie mit einem Beitrag von Dr. phil. Riwkah Schärf. 1948.

KERÉNYI, KARL: *Die Antike Religion*. 1940.

Prometheus. 1946.

Niobe. 1949.

KNIGHT, G. WILSON: *Chariot of Wrath*. 1942.

LANGTON, EDWARD: *Satan. A Portrait*. A study of the character of Satan through all the ages. 1945.

LEEUW, G. VAN DER: *La Religion dans son Essence et ses Manifestations: Phénomélogie de la Religion*. 1948.

LEWIS, C. S.: *A Preface to Paradise Lost*. 1942.
LOVEJOY, A. O.: *Essays in the History of Ideas*. 1948.
MASSON, DAVID: *The Three Devils and other Essays*. 1874.
MCCOLLEY, GRANT: 'Paradise Lost', *Harv. Theol. Rev.* xxxii. 1939.
MCLACHLAN, H.: *The Religious Opinions of Milton, Locke and Newton*. 1941.
MARTIN, L. C.: 'Shakespeare, Lucretius and the Commonplaces'. *R.E.S.* xxi. 1945.
MUSGROVE, S.: 'Is the Devil an Ass?' *R.E.S.* xxi. 1945.
MUTSCHMANN, H.: *Der andere Milton*. 1920.
'Studies concerning the origin of Paradise Lost'. *Acta et Commutationes, etc.* Dorpat. 1924.
NEUMANN, ERICH: *Ursprungsgeschichte des Bewusstseins*. 1949.
OSTROWSKI-SACHS, MARGARETE: 'Die Wandlungen des Prometheus-Mythus. *Der Psychologe*, ii. 1950.
OSGOOD, C. G.: *The Classical Mythology of Milton's English Poems*. 1900.
PICCARD, CH.: *Les Religions Préhelléniques*. 1948.
PRAZ, MARIO: *The Romantic Agony*. 1933.
RĂJAN, B.: 'Simple, Sensuous and Passionate. *R.E.S.* xxi. 1945.
Paradise Lost and the Seventeenth-century Reader. 1947.
RALEIGH, WALTER: *Milton*. 1900.
ROSCHER: *Lexicon der Griechischen und Römischen Mythologie*.
ROSS, M. M.: *Milton's Royalism: A Study of the Conflit of Symbol and Idea in the Poems*. 1943.
RUSSELL, BERTRAND: *History of Western Philosophy*. 1946.
SAINT-VICTOR, PAUL DE: *Les deux Masques*. 3rd ed. 1883.
SAURAT, DENIS: *Milton: Man and Thinker*. 1925.
SCHÄRF, RIWKAH: 'Die Gestalt des Satans im Alten Testament', in Jung: *Symbolik des Geistes*. 1948.
SEWELL, ARTHUR: *A Study of Milton's Christian Doctrine*. 1939.
SIEBERT, TH.: 'Untersuchungen über Miltons Kunst vom psychologischen Standpunktaus'. *Anglia* liv. 1930.
SMITH, LOGAN PEARSELL: *Milton and his Modern Critics*. 1940.
STOLL, E. E.: *Poets and Playwrights*. 1930.
'Give the Devil his Due: a reply to Mr. Lewis'. *R.E.S.* xx. 1944.
TEMPLE, WILLIAM: *The Genius of English Poetry*. 1939.
THOMSON, G.: *Aeschylus: The Prometheus Bound*, edited with Introduction, Commentary and Translation by George Thomson. 1932.
TILLYARD, E. W. M.: *Milton*. 1930.
VOLZ, PAUL: *Das Dämonische in Jahwe*. 1924.
WALDOCK, A. J. A.: *Paradise Lost and its Critics*. 1947.
WARNER, REX: *Prometheus Bound*. 1947.
WILLEY, BASIL: *The Seventeenth-century Background*. 1934.
WILLIAMS, CHARLES: Introduction to the World's Classics edition of Milton's *English Poems*. 1940.
WRIGHT, B. A.: 'Review of Mr. Lewis' *Preface*' in *R.E.S.* xx. 1944.

INDEX

INDEX

INDEX